An Introduction to the U.S. Health Care System

Second Edition

D0701417

MILTON I. ROEMER has been a Professor at the School of Public Health of the University of California, Los Angeles, since 1962. He taught previously at the Cornell University Institute of Hospital Administration (1957–61) and at Yale Medical School (1949–51). Dr. Roemer earned the M.D. degree in 1940 and also holds master's degrees in sociology and in public health.

Dr. Roemer has served at all levels of health administration—as a County Health Officer in West Virginia, a state and provincial health official in New Jersey and Saskatchewan, Canada, a commissioned officer of the U.S. Public Health Service in Washington, and a Section Chief of the World Health Organization headquarters in Geneva, Switzerland. In 1974 he was elected to the Institute of Medicine of the National Academy of Sciences.

As a consultant to international agencies, Dr. Roemer has studied health care organization in 58 countries on all the continents. He is the author of 30 books and over 350 articles on the social aspects of medicine. In 1977, he was the recipient of the American Public Health Association International Award for Excellence in Promoting and Protecting the Health of People. In 1983, the APHA awarded Dr. Roemer its highest honor, the Sedgwick Memorial Medal for Distinguished Service in Public Health.

An Introduction to the U.S. Health Care System

Second Edition

Milton I. Roemer, M.D.

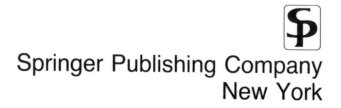

Springer Publishing Company
New York

Springer Publishing Company, Inc.
536 Broadway
New York, New York 10012

86 87 88 89 90 / 5 4 3 2 1

Library of Congress Cataloging-in-Publication Data

Roemer, Milton Irwin
   An introduction to the U.S. health care system.

   Includes bibliographies and index.
   1. Medical care—United States. I. Title.
[DNLM: 1. Health Services—United States. W 84 AA1 R7i]
RA395.A3R626   1985   362.1'0973   85-26131
ISBN 0-8261-3983-3 (pbk.)

Chapter 2 is based on an article entitled "Prospects of Ambulatory Health Care and Their Meaning for Allied Health Personnel" by Milton I. Roemer, *New York University Education Quarterly*, *14*(3–4):17–22, Spring–Summer 1983. Used by permission.

Chapter 3 is reprinted from "The Politics of Public Health in the United States" by Milton I. Roemer. In Theodor J. Litman and Leonard S. Robins (Eds.), *Health Politics and Policy*, pp. 261–273. Copyright © 1984 by John Wiley & Sons, New York. Used by permission.

Chapter 5 is based on an article entitled "The Value of Medical Care for Health Promotion" by Milton I. Roemer. In *American Journal of Public Health*, *74*(3):243–248, March 1984. Used by permission.

Chapter 6 is adapted from "The Social Consequences of Free Trade in Health Care: A Public Health Response to Orthodox Economics" by John E. Roemer and Milton I. Roemer. In *International Journal of Health Services*, *12*(1):111–129. © 1982. Used by permission.

Chapter 7 is based on an article entitled "I.S. Falk, the Committee on the Costs of Medical Care, and the Drive for National Health Insurance" by Milton I. Roemer. In *American Journal of Public Health*, *75*(8):841–848, August 1985.

Chapter 8 is reprinted, by permission of the World Health Orgnization, from Milton I. Roemer, "Medical Ethics and Education for Social Responsibility," *World Health Forum*, *3*(4):357–375, 1982.

Printed in the United States of America

Contents

Chapter 3

The Development of Public Health in the United States   49

Chapter 4

Nursing and Developments in Other Health Professions   67

Chapter 5

Integration of Medical Care and Health Promotion   85

Preface to the Second Edition

The Preface to the first edition of this book, published in 1982, begins as follows:

> Arrangements for health services in the United States, compared with other countries, are very complex. They are bewildering to most Americans who seek care for some health problem, and even to persons engaged within the health care system. A nurse or doctor or pharmacist or laboratory technician may know and perform his or her functions very well, but still have little understanding of their relationships to all other parts of the system. To foreign visitors, American health services are particularly confusing.
>
> This book is intended to clarify the basic structure and operations of the U.S. health care system. By approaching the system *as a whole* and drawing its contours with broad strokes, this account attempts to simplify a picture which otherwise may seem like a jigsaw puzzle.

In the first edition, the health services were described as the products of an "industry," which required the input of certain resources, economic support, and so on. Unfortunately, in recent years the entrepreneurial aspects of health care have become all too prominent, and commercialization has begun to challenge the concept of health care as a social or human right—a concept long accepted in the United Nations, the World Health Organization, and elsewhere. In this edition, therefore, we shall avoid the inappropriate reference to health services as an "industry."

The health care system, of course, has a structure and dynamics that can be analyzed in an orderly way. Like other systems in society, it has a complex organizational structure, usually analyzed as "programs," one of which is the private market. It has arrangements for the production of resources (manpower, facilities, etc.), and it has numerous sources of economic support. There are various methods of management of the system, including planning, regulation, and other processes of control. All these system attributes lead to diverse patterns for the delivery of health services. This general analysis of the U.S. health care system is offered in Chapter 1.

All the other chapters examine special aspects of the health care system in greater depth—by historical development, by greater analysis of current circumstances, or by both of these approaches. In Chapter 2, we focus on the delivery of one type of health service, ambulatory care, which until recently has been relatively slow to respond to social needs. This chapter explores the different ways that ambulatory health services have been organized, under diverse sponsorships, in order to meet the needs of special populations or disorders in American society.

Controversy has long marked the development of the content and scope of public health services in the United States. These services have typically been provided by government agencies—local, state, and federal—so that inevitably their development has been entangled with general political issues on the "proper" role of government in a free enterprise economic system. While health responsibilities have been assigned to many other branches of government, public health agencies have extended their range of functions much beyond their initial confinement to preventive services. These developments are reviewed in Chapter 3.

Chapter 4 is devoted to nursing and selected aspects of other health professions. Nurses are the most numerous of the health professionals, and continued change has marked their mode of education and the definition of their functions. The development of health manpower in general and of nursing in particular reflects the issues and adjustments occurring in the entire U.S. health care system.

In Chapters 5 and 6, we enter somewhat deeper waters. Chapter 5 reviews the main accomplishments of disease prevention and also of medical care, and considers some of the subtleties of social policy concerned with relationships between these two major approaches to health. Chapter 6 examines a major tenet of contemporary social policy—the free market and competition—and poses questions on the applicability of this tenet to the health care system of the United States. What are the implications and consequences of the classical economic market for the provision and utilization of health services?

In the United States, many years of study and controversy have concerned the problems of financing medical care, developing voluntary health insurance, and shaping legislation to insure the entire population against medical care costs. In 1922 the Committee on the Costs of Medical Care fired the opening shot in these long battles, and the main story is told in Chapter 7.

Finally, in Chapter 8, we explore the role that ethical precepts have played in health care systems of the United States and also in other countries. We examine to what extent "medical ethics" have been concerned with the welfare of populations, as distinguished from the relationships between individual doctors and patients. The requirements of a truly social code of ethics are explored in the complex modern world of health services.

This volume is intentionally brief. Almost any topic mentioned would have to be elaborated on in much greater detail if specific changes were to be sought in the structure or function of American health services. The literature on the U.S. health care system is abundant, and the references at the end of most of the chapters will guide the reader who wishes to examine certain subjects in greater depth. It is hoped that this introductory text will serve to clarify the main contours of the U.S. health care system and to shed some additional light on certain aspects that have acquired special significance in the contemporary scene.

Milton I. Roemer, M.D.

Chapter 1

The Health Care System as a Whole

The health care system of any country can be analyzed in different ways, but this account of the U.S. system will be based on a model found useful in comparative studies. Thus, every system of health care has five main components, the relationships among which may be illustrated as follows:

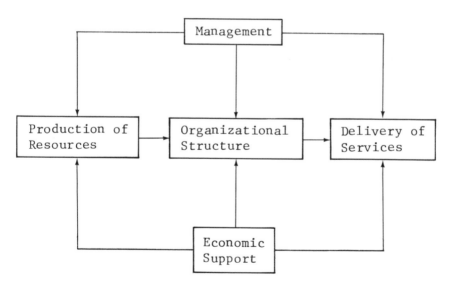

MAJOR FEATURES OF THE U.S. SYSTEM

In the perspective of the world's 160 nations, the U.S. system of health care embodies several major features. First, since the United States is an affluent industrialized country, its health care system has abundant resources, and it spends a great deal of money. Second, since this is a federated nation, the governance of the system is highly decentralized to numerous states, counties, and communities. Third, since this nation has a free market economy, very permissive laissez-faire concepts are incorporated throughout its health care system. These concepts are apparent in the forms taken by all five system components shown in the above figure.

All three of these system characteristics are relative—that is, relative to the policies and practices of other countries. There are, of course, other affluent and industrialized nations, other federated republics, and other laissez-faire economies. The degree of these attributes in the U.S. health care system, however, is especially great. They have resulted in a system which is remarkably pluralistic and complex, with very different meanings for various sections of its population.

The federated political structure can be traced to the American Revolution against the British monarchy, and the determination to avoid strong central government. Even within the central government, there are "checks and balances" among the executive, legislative, and judicial branches, which restrain governmental actions of all types. The free market economy was emerging in Europe in the early nineteenth century, just when the "new world" was beginning to develop. Inevitably the American health care system was influenced by these dynamic economic processes around it.

Yet the U.S. health care system, like that of all countries, is not static. In spite of the dedication of national and health professional leaders to free market principles, many interventions in the operation of the market have been necessary. As the expectations of people for recovery from disease and for the maintenance of good health have risen, more initiatives have become necessary to change the contours of all five system components. Social actions have been taken to increase the quantity and quality of resources produced, to plan and modify system management, to alter the overall system structure, to strengthen mechanisms of economic support, and to rationalize and improve the delivery of services. The resultant profile of the U.S. health care system today will be examined below.

THE HEALTH OF THE U.S. POPULATION

For reasons that far transcend the health care system, the U.S. population as a whole is among the healthiest of the world's large nations. Within its 240,000,000 population, however, there are great inequalities, and much of the excellent health service of which the nation is capable has not been made accessible to everyone.

Examining first the overall picture, life expectancy for U.S. residents was 74.5 years at birth, as of 1982. The difference is substantial for the sexes, it being 70.8 years for men and 78.2 years for women. More indicative of differences in the standard of living, as well as health services, is the contrast of life expectancies for white and black races. On the whole, blacks suffer disadvantages in virtually every condition affecting health; their life expectancy at birth is 69.5 years (as of 1982), compared with 75.1 years for whites.

The U.S. infant mortality rate in 1982 was 11.2 per 1000 live births. While this, of course, is low, it is slightly higher than that of some 15 other countries—mostly in Western Europe, but also including Canada, Japan, and the German Democratic Republic. It is perhaps significant that these countries have less wealth than the United States (as measured by gross national product per capita), but they all have systems of national health care which make services freely accessible (or nearly free) to virtually everyone.

Tuberculosis and other serious infectious diseases have been greatly reduced in the United States. The leading causes of death are the noninfectious disorders that are prevalent in the later years of life, followed by deaths due to violence. Adjusting disease-specific death rates for the nation's age composition in 1940, the leading causes of death in 1982 were:

Cause	Deaths per 100,000
Diseases of the heart	190.8
Malignant neoplasms	133.3
Accidents and adverse effects	37.1
Cerebrovascular diseases	36.1
Suicide	11.5
Pneumonia and influenza	11.3
Chronic liver disease and cirrhosis	10.4
Homicide and legal intervention	9.7
Diabetes mellitus	9.2
All causes	556.4

A great cause for optimism in the United States has been the trend of heart disease mortality during the last 30 years. After increasing since 1900 (when satisfactory records were first kept), in 1950 the *age-adjusted* death rate from diseases of the heart began to decline. It fell from 307.6 deaths per 100,000 population in 1950 to 190.8 in 1982. (The manifest increase in observable cases was due, of course, to the rising proportion of people living to older age levels.) The exact causes of this trend are not clear, but it is likely that both improvements in medical care and modifications in living habits (diet, smoking, exercise, etc.) have had impacts. This experience has given great impetus to a movement for greater emphasis on prevention and health promotion, and encouragement of healthful lifestyles in the U.S. health care system.

The United States is one of the few countries to tabulate data regularly on morbidity from all causes in general populations; this is based on periodic household interviews of a nationwide sample of the civilian and noninstitutionalized population. Of various measures used, the broadest is the number of "restricted activity days" per person per year. (This indicator identifies any disorder in a worker, a school child, a housewife, or anyone else.) In 1981, there were found to be 18.5 restricted activity days per person per year in the United States. The differences by family income were striking:

Family Income Per Year	Restricted-activity Days per Person per Year
Less than $7,000	32.1
$7,000–$9,999	23.5
$10,000–$14,999	18.1
$15,000–$24,999	16.2
$25,000 or more	13.6

A reflection of the dynamics of the U.S. health care system is to consider the contacts with physicians, as well as inpatient hospital days, per person per year in families of different incomes. In 1981, these relationships were as follows:

Family Income per Year	Physician Contacts	Hospital Days
Less than $7,000	5.6	1.32
$7,000–$9,999	4.9	1.16
$10,000–$14,999	4.5	1.06
$15,000–$24,999	4.5	0.84
$25,000 or more	4.4	0.77

Thus, the lower income groups—in accordance with their higher rate of morbidity shown above—have contacts with doctors slightly more often than the higher income groups. Nevertheless, for reasons probably related to their general conditions of living, they end up receiving higher rates of hospital care. Thirty years ago, data showed the lower income groups to have higher rates of illness, as they have still, but lower rates of contact with both physicians and hospitals than the upper income groups. The health care system, in other words, has evidently improved in its degree of equity, but not sufficiently to overcome the generally unhealthful effects of an environment of deprivation or poverty.

THE ORGANIZATIONAL STRUCTURE

To present and analyze the U.S. health care system today, it is most enlightening to begin with an account of its organizational structure. This component stands at the center of the system model, pictured earlier, like the trunk of a tree. Then we may consider the four other components that contribute to or support this organizational structure, and how the whole combination of relationships differ from those in other national systems.

The organizational structure of a health care system is often described in terms of an array of various "health programs." The forms and proportionate role of each program differ greatly among national systems. In the United States, as in most countries, however, some five major types of health program operate to some degree. They may be analyzed as the principal governmental health authority, other agencies of government with health functions, voluntary health agencies, enterprises with health functions, and the private health care market. The size, shape, and proportions of these programs define the organizational structure of the U.S. health care system.

The Principal Governmental Health Authority

In most countries, there is a central governmental authority that carries major responsibility for the health protection of the population. In some countries, this responsibility is carried along with other major responsibilities, and this is the arrangement in the permissive health care system of the United States. Until recently, the U.S. government's equivalent to a Ministry of Health was combined with authority for other major fields in a Department of Health, Education, and Welfare. Not long ago responsibility for education was withdrawn, but the Department of Health and Human Services is now responsible for the nation's massive programs of social security and public assistance, as well as those for most aspects of health. Within this Department there is a vast organizational structure handling the responsibilities of the U.S. federal government in health resource development, health services, health research, health care financing, health planning and regulation, and other governmental functions within the national health care system.

We need not explore in detail the organization and functions of the U.S. Department of Health and Human Services; here it may simply be noted that most of the Department's responsibilities are fulfilled by allocation of money and delegation of authority to numerous other public and private entities throughout the nation. Because this country is a federation of states, the U.S. Constitution grants the states a great deal of autonomy and responsibility in all social affairs, including health. There are relatively few health functions carried out directly from the national level (principally by the U.S. Public Health Service within the Department of HHS), such as health examination of immigrants, regulation of drugs that move in interstate commerce, special epidemiological investigations, compilation of national health statistics, and medical services to American Indians.

Below the national level, in each of the 50 states there is likewise a major health agency, although sometimes it also is combined with authorities for social welfare or other functions. The administrative configuration and scope of functions of the state health agencies are highly variable. The heads of these agencies are ordinarily appointed by an elected governor; they are responsible entirely to the state governor and not at all to the national health authority. Only insofar as certain standards must be met, as a condition for receipt of certain national grants, must the state accept national direction. Federal grants for hospital construction, for example, require that the state must have a law on licensure of hospitals; wide leeway is allowed, however, in the provisions of such laws. Similarly, below the level of state government, there are units of local government—counties and cities or sometimes special districts—that also have a major health agency, which likewise has great autonomy. On certain health matters, the local health department may carry out functions delegated by the state agency, but on most matters it has full authority within the constraints of the general local government.

Other Agencies of Government with Health Functions

Most governmental structures are determined by historical developments. Public health agencies grew out of recognition of the need to protect people from hazards of the environment and of epidemic diseases; these were dangers to the entire population. Social insurance, however, was a movement to protect the economic position of low-paid workers, who could be ruined by the costs of sickness—costs referable to lost earnings and also to needed medical care. Almost everywhere, therefore, the place of social insurance in the structure of government has been different from that of public health.

In the United States, we have discussed the federal Department of Health and Human Services, and within it the U.S. Public Health Service. The first national social insurance program to finance medical care, however, was placed administratively in the Social Security Administration, not the Public Health Service—that is, Medicare insurance for the aged, enacted in 1965. Even when the Medicare program was later withdrawn from the Social Security Administration and combined with the public assistance program of Medicaid for health care of the poor, it was placed in still another organizational setting, the Health Care Financing Administration. Several other agencies of the federal government in the United States also administer important health programs. The Department of Labor, with its Occupational Safety and Health Administration, has the main responsibility for protecting the health of workers at their places of work. The health and safety of miners, however, is a concern of the Bureau of Mines in the Department of the Interior. Many aspects of the health of agricultural families and farm workers, including control of the diseases of animals, are a concern of the Department of Agriculture. For certain historical reasons, the control of narcotic drugs has long been in the Department of Treasury. The Veterans Administration is an independent federal authority which, among other things, is responsible for the operation of the nation's largest network of public hospitals—those for military veterans, whether or not their disorders are connected with military service. The separate branches of the armed forces, as in nearly all countries, operate their own large subsystems of health services in time of peace as well as war, under the federal Department of Defense. Even the Department of Justice is responsible for health facilities in a network of federal prisons.

At the state and local levels in the United States, the multiplicity of governmental agencies concerned with health is even greater. The organizational layout is not the same in any two states. In most states, the medical care programs for the poor—defined in various ways—come under departments of social welfare or public assistance. Factory inspection for accident or disease hazards is usually a function of state departments of labor or industry. Worker's compensation programs—to help workers who incur work-connected injuries or diseases—are responsible for much medical care and rehabilitation; they are generally under the control of other special commissions or agencies. Programs of vocational rehabilitation are often within state departments of education, although a major part of their task is medical. Special state authorities are usually concerned with the licensure of doctors, nurses, pharmacists, and other health personnel. Public water supply and sewage disposal systems are the responsibility of separate departments of public works in many states, and in most states there are special authorities established for the control of air and stream pollution. Even the overall planning of health services is often assigned by governors to a special agency other than the State Department of Health.

At the local level, the dispersion of governmental health responsibilities in the United States is generally as great. Local boards and agencies concerned with welfare (of the poor and disabled), with public schools, with garbage disposal, with water and sanitation, with local government hospitals, with first-aid in emergencies, with mental health services, with parks and recreation, and with other programs having health aspects function separately from the local Department of Health. Only a handful of America's 3100 counties have developed integration of these many health functions under one major local health agency.

Voluntary Agencies

In all countries there are nongovernmental agencies that play a role in health care systems. Known commonly as voluntary agencies, they have arisen for various reasons: to perform a service not being rendered by government, to pursue a certain objective with special vigor and dedication in order to attain it sooner, to advance or protect the interests of a certain population group, and sometimes even to carry out certain tasks at the behest of official bodies. The term "voluntary agency" is applied ordinarily to such organizations that are not conducting a business for profit and hence are nonprofit.

In the United States, the permissive character of the health care system is vividly demonstrated in the enormous multiplicity of voluntary health agencies. There are hundreds of agencies that raise funds and carry out programs for fighting certain diseases—cancer, tuberculosis, mental illness, and the like. Other agencies focus on the health of certain population groups—children, American Indians, war veterans, and so on. Still other voluntary agencies are concerned with certain types of health service, such as visiting nurse care, hospitalization, or blood donations. The voluntary agency may be devoted exclusively to health purposes, or health services may be incidental to certain larger purposes, such as those of church groups or religious missions (domestically or abroad).

Most numerous in the United States are the disease-specific voluntary agencies that mobilize the interest and financial contributions of millions of citizens. The American Cancer Society is illustrative. As cancer has come to affect more people and has become the second highest cause of death, large numbers of people have become deeply concerned about solving the riddle of this complex disease and helping its victims. Although initiated in a few large cities, there soon was formed a national organization, with branches in every state of the nation. Below the state level, there are city or county chapters. Funds are raised from individual donors locally, and a percentage of these is passed along to the national headquarters. A large share of the national funds is used for supporting research projects. Funds kept at the local level are sometimes used to support "cancer detection clinics" or to provide compassionate services to terminal cancer patients. The local, state, and national units of disease-specific voluntary agencies in the

United States number in the tens of thousands. In the long run, the initiative taken by voluntary health agencies has often stimulated governmental bodies to do similar work.

Nongovernmental associations of professional health personnel must be counted as another type of voluntary agency. Their funds are raised by membership dues, rather than donations, and their activities are focused largely on advancing the interests of their members. This may be through programs of continuing education and various strategies to elevate professional standards. At the same time, much of the effort of bodies like the American Medical Association or the American Dental Association is devoted to opposing legislative proposals that are regarded as threatening the independence and economic positions of these professional groups.

Enterprises with Health Functions

Enterprises are relevant to the structure of health care systems in two ways: first, insofar as the establishment provides certain health services to its employees, and second, when the enterprise is commercially engaged in the provision of health service or carrying out some other function in a health care system.

In the United States, in-plant health services are generally of very limited scope, except in large establishments (with more than 500 workers or thereabout). In smaller factories, services are usually limited to first-aid by an industrial nurse or perhaps only a medicine chest available to the workers. Large plants or mines may maintain a staff of physicians and nurses who perform periodic and preplacement examinations, treat any intercurrent illness, whether or not job-connected, and promote education for healthful living. Enterprises in isolated locations, such as railroad junctions or lumber mills, may sometimes operate comprehensive medical care programs for workers. Industrial firms, of course, are obligated by law to protect workers from accidents and occupational diseases, although enforcement is often weak.

With respect to enterprises involved in the health sector as their main commercial objective, these play an especially large part in the U.S. health care system. In connection with resource production, pharmaceutical companies are very important. Along with them are the manufacturers of x-ray and laboratory equipment, surgical instruments and supplies, orthopedic appliances, eyeglasses, hearing aids, dental prostheses, and so on. Relevant to insurance for the costs of medical care (discussed below under economic support), hundreds of companies are engaged in the sale of a vast range of insurance policies financing various "packages" of hospital, medical, and related services. (The nonprofit Blue Cross and Blue Shield insurance organizations should probably be counted among voluntary health agencies.) Also, a rising proportion of U.S. general hospitals are coming under the control of for-profit firms—facilities with some 12 percent of the general beds available in the early 1980s. Nursing homes for the aged and chronically ill have long been predominantly proprietary, with 80 percent of their beds in units operated for profit.

The Private Market

As the residual part of the organizational structure of any health care system, the arrangements of a private market for medical care are important in most countries. One may regard the "private sector" in social systems from the vantage point of the buyer or the seller, or in the context of health services from the vantage point of the source of financing or that of the provider of services. Here, in considering the system's organizational structure, we take the viewpoint of the seller or how the services are provided. (Later, in discussing economic support, we will consider financing from the viewpoint of the buyer.)

From the vantage point of health care provision, the U.S. health care system is overwhelmingly dominated by a private market. The great majority of providers of health service are in private business, as of the 1980s, even though system trends have been changing many of these relationships. Ambulatory medical care (both general and specialized), dental care, pharmacy services, medical and surgical services in hospitals, optical services, fitting of prosthetic appliances—all these services are furnished predominantly by private practitioners. The personal preventive services may be provided often by governmental or other organized entities, but even a substantial share of these is given by private providers. It is especially noteworthy that, even when the financial support for health services has been collectivized, as in the various public or voluntary health insurance programs or in the tax-supported Medicaid program for the poor, the provision of services remains substantially a process in the private market. For care in the doctor's private office, this is quite obvious, but even in a hospitalized case, the service is rendered to a private patient, and any responsible "third-party" agency pays essentially a private fee.

Over recent decades there has been a prominent trend for U.S. physicians to join together in groups of different sizes for many technical, economic, and professional reasons. Close to half of the American physicians who practice outside of institutions are in groups of three or more, working with nurses and numerous allied personnel. The solo practitioner is gradually disappearing. The vast majority of these group-practice doctors, nevertheless, function as private practitioners, even though they share their incomes in some way. The provision of dental care is similarly delivered from a private market setting for the vast bulk of services rendered. The same applies to the dispensing of drugs and other services.

The hospital care of short-term patients, on the other hand, is provided principally by nonprofit or governmental facilities (although we have noted that even this is changing). Insofar as certain physicians work full time in hospitals—as residents in training or as full-time specialists in certain fields, mainly pathology and radiology—they may be salaried employees and not in private practice. This pattern has also been growing, but the lion's share of medical or surgical services to patients in American hospitals is still provided by private practitioners.

PRODUCTION OF RESOURCES

The operation of health programs in the organizational structure of every national system of health care depends on the availability of many resources. In the main these consist of health manpower, health facilities, various commodities (including drugs), and knowledge. All four types of resources must be produced, deployed, and used. What are the ways that this is done in the United States, starting with the health manpower?

Health Manpower

The oldest form of health personnel is the physician, who is found to some extent in every health care system of the world. Everywhere physicians are trained in special schools or institutes, which usually play a general policy role in health care systems, beyond their educational functions. In the United States there are numerous medical colleges—about 125 or one per 1,840,000 people. All but a few are attached to universities, where they are separate colleges, sometimes loosely linked with other professional schools as "centers of health sciences." About half of these institutions are sponsored by state governments, as part of state public universities, and half are under private auspices. All of the schools, however, have received substantial financial support from the federal government for many years. Entry to U.S. medical schools usually requires a university bachelor's degree (requiring four years of study), and medical schooling requires another four years, making eight academic years. Virtually all 50 states also require an internship in a hospital for at least one year, so that medical qualification involves a total of nine years after secondary school. Admission to medical schools is selective, and only about half of those who apply are accepted.

The vast majority of U.S. medical students must pay high tuitions, although these tend to be higher in the private than in the public schools; for a small percentage of students there are fellowships and loan programs which may help to meet the costs of tuition and living expenses. For a very small fraction of students, federal or state public subsidy programs finance the entire costs of medical schooling on the condition that the graduate serves in a designated area of doctor-shortage (usually rural) for a period equivalent to the years of subsidy. After academic training, when the young doctor is interning, he/she has all living expenses met by the hospital and is paid a modest salary. The vast majority of interns proceed to further training for qualification as specialists, and as specialty residents they are usually paid attractive salaries. Some 85 percent of active U.S. physicians currently have such specialty credentials.

The optimal supply of physicians required to meet the health needs of a country has long been a subject of discussion and debate. In a period of economic difficulties, such as during the worldwide depression of 1929–1939, there was widespread opinion about a "surplus" of doctors. Then, when economic conditions are favorable and social insurance facilitates financial access to medical care, physicians become very busy and a "shortage" is perceived. Thus, in the permissive United States health care system, there were about 150 doctors per 100,000 population in 1900–1910. This ratio then declined or remained stationary until World War II. By the end of the war (1945) a serious shortage was felt, and both federal and state governments gave grants for strengthening the medical schools, both public and private. By 1980 there were more than 200 active physicians per 100,000 and the supply was continuing to increase. In the early 1980s, it was again widely believed that too many doctors were being produced (although not everyone shared this view).

In the affluent United States, there were 586 registered nurses per 100,000 population in 1982, plus about 240 per 100,000 vocational nurses. Until about 1965, the vast majority of these young women (and some men) were prepared in hospital-based nursing schools requiring three years of training. Then a different educational pattern, which had started earlier, gained momentum—the preparation of professional nurses through two years of academic study in community colleges. By 1980 the vast majority of registered nurses in the United States were being trained through these academic courses lasting two years; practical experience was acquired principally after they became employed. As in several other professions in this country, nursing leadership sought continuous upgrading, and university-based programs also developed, turning out nurses with bachelor's degrees.

The heterogeneity of the U.S. health care system has created a need for nurses in many types of service. Although the majority of registered nurses work in hospitals (61 percent in 1977), some 39 percent work in nursing homes for the chronically ill, in public health agencies, in schools, in industrial clinics, in nursing education, in private medical or dental offices, in private duty positions, and in other settings. The turnover among registered nurses is very high in the United States, since many leave nursing service after a few years for other types of employment or marriage.

In some countries, pharmacies are devoted almost exclusively to the sale of drugs, so that the numbers of pharmacists produced are relatively smaller than in countries where the "drugstore" sells also candy, tobacco products, and many other commodities. Thus, in the United States there are 68 pharmacists per 100,000 population. In Great Britain, where the "chemist shop" dispenses solely drugs, there are only 28 pharmacists per 100,000.

The numbers and functions of dental personnel in the various health care systems is an interesting reflection of system policies. In the permissive system of the United States, there are 52 dentists per 100,000 population. There are numerous dental hygienists and dental assistants, but their functions are restricted essentially to preventive work or to assisting the dentist at the chairside; publicly financed clinics for dental care are scarce.

Health Facilities

In the United States, with its permissive health care system, the total hospital bed supply in 1981 was 6.0 beds per 100,000 population, of which 4.4 beds per 1000 were in short-stay general hospitals. In the cooperative-type health care systems of Western Europe, with national health care programs, the hospital bed supplies are usually greater.

The supply of beds in a health care system does not necessarily reflect the volume of hospitalization provided to the people. This depends upon how fully the available beds are used (the occupancy rate), the average length of stay per case, and other factors. Thus, although the United States has a lesser supply of general hospital beds per 1000 than several countries with cooperative health care systems, the U.S. rate of admissions to general hospitals in 1982 was quite high—158.5 per 1000 persons per year—and the average length of stay quite short. In France, with a much greater general bed supply, the corresponding admission rate was 167.8 per 1000 per year, and in Sweden the admission rate was 164.1 per 1000 per year—with appreciably longer average stays per case.

The ownership or sponsorship of the nation's 7100 hospitals is another important characteristic, reflecting how the institutions function. In general, hospitals owned by government serve patients according to their health needs, while those under nongovernmental ownership usually impose charges for their use. These charges are often paid by insurance, but the patient must then have insurance coverage. There are many other implications to hospital sponsorship, but as a general rule the services of hospitals under government are distributed in more equitable relationship to health needs than the services of privately owned hospitals, whether the latter are sponsored by nonprofit (voluntary) or for-profit (proprietary) organizations. Governmental hospitals may belong to any level of government—national, provincial, or local.

In the United States, as of 1981, only 27 percent of the general short-stay hospital beds were in institutions owned by governmental agencies; this excluded mental hospitals, which are overwhelmingly controlled by state governments. Among the 73 percent of general hospital beds that are privately sponsored, 65 percent are under the auspices of nonprofit bodies (both religious and nonsectarian) and 8 percent are proprietary (for profit). In the late 1970s and the 1980s, however, a growing proportion of hospitals came under the control of for-profit corporations. This increasing "corporatization" or commercialization of American health services has been a source of mounting concern among many medical leaders.

In all types of health care system, hospitals operate outpatient departments, for the diagnosis and treatment of patients not necessarily requiring bed care. The relative importance of outpatient departments (OPDs) is greater in most other countries than in the United States, because they are a principal setting for consultation with specialists—not just by the poor but by all persons. Beyond the OPD, however, a major organized resource for the provision of ambulatory care in nearly all countries of the world is the health center. Its character and role, nevertheless, differ substantially among the various types of health care system.

In the entrepreneurial and permissive setting of the United States, health centers were first established in the 1920s as facilities for coordinated provision of preventive services—often by separate agencies for promotion of maternal and child health, for the control of tuberculosis, for hygienic education, and the like. They later came to house official public health agencies. Attempts to extend their scope to provision of medical treatment of the poor were successfully resisted by private physicians, on the ground that this would constitute improper invasion of the sphere of private medicine. Not until the 1960s was the role of the health center in the United States broadened to include general ambulatory medical care for selected population groups. Very poor families in urban slums were the main beneficiaries, but special units—often called simply clinics—were established for migratory farm workers, for residents of blighted Appalachian areas, for low-income children and youths, for American Indians, and for others. Special government subsidies supported these health centers under various federal laws.

The health centers just described limit their services essentially to primary health care, including both its preventive and therapeutic aspects. Another important type of free-standing facility in the United States is the private group practice clinic, in which a number of doctors, usually of different specialties, join together as a team to provide a broad range of ambulatory services. In 1975 there were some 7700 of these private units, far more than the approximately 1000 health centers supported by governmental grants. Other facilities for organized ambulatory care are focused on industrial workers (supported by management) and on school children (supported usually by educational authorities), but these are devoted essentially to prevention and case detection. Public health agencies, of course, also sponsor clinics for venereal disease control (including treatment) and dental care of children, and in recent years some of these clinics have broadened their scope to include general primary care.

Health Commodities

A third essential type of health resource in any health care system is a wide variety of commodities. These include all sorts of equipment for the diagnosis and treatment of disease, supplies for prevention as well as treatment, prosthetic appliances including eyeglasses and hearing aids, dental prostheses, and, perhaps most important, drugs.

Drugs in the economically developed countries are, with few exceptions, produced by pharmaceutical companies on a large scale, and then distributed to the population through large numbers of pharmacies or general health care facilities (hospitals and health centers). In the permissive health care system of the United States, the pharmaceutical industry contains hundreds of firms, although about 20 major companies sell most of the products. Newly discovered or invented drugs are protected by patents (which endure for 17 years) so that they are sold under "brand names," which may command high prices. After a patent expires, the drug's nonpatented or "generic name" may be used to identify the product sold by any manufacturer.

With many companies engaged in drug manufacturing, there is much competition and a great deal of advertising to win the preferences of physicians. There may be, for example, scores or hundreds of different drugs to combat insomnia and induce sleep, often with very little difference among them—sometimes no difference except their names and perhaps their color or packaging. It has been estimated that more than 25 percent of the price paid by the pharmacist for drugs is referrable to the manufacturer's advertising costs. On top of this, the patient must pay the "middleman" costs of the pharmacist and sometimes a wholesale distributor. Although competition may breed extravagant claims for a particular drug, on several occasions drug firms have been found guilty of collusion to fix prices at a specified high level in violation of the U.S. antitrust laws.

Regulations in the United States indicate which drugs may be dispensed only with a doctor's prescription and which may be sold "over-the-counter" directly to patients. In 1930, three-quarters of the U.S. expenditures on drugs were for the latter type, often called patent medicines, but in 1980 these relationships were reversed. Drug therapy over the years has become increasingly effective, and prescription prices have risen steeply—even though not so steeply as hospital charges. The development of antibiotic drugs that can effectively combat most infectious diseases (including tuberculosis, syphilis, and gonorrhea), drugs to reduce hypertension, to combat the most serious manifestations of psychosis, to treat diabetes, to eliminate the pains of gout and arthritis, to reduce the eye pressure that leads to glaucoma, to extend the life of patients with cancer—all these have greatly advanced the effectiveness of medical practice in affluent countries like the United States. Even greater benefits have probably come from the many vaccines discovered and produced for the prevention of infectious diseases, such as diphtheria, poliomyelitis, and measles.

Yet the enormous multiplicity of drug preparations in a permissive free enterprise setting has also created problems. The large expenditures on advertising have been noted, and this includes the advertising both of prescription or "legend" drugs to doctors and of nonprescription drugs directly to the general population. The numbers and attributes of different drugs are so great that the average physician could not possibly be expected to remember them all, especially as hundreds of new products appear on the market each year. American pharmacies, which must each respond to the prescription orders of numerous doctors, must keep on hand enormous stocks of diverse products, which is very costly. To get around this problem, many hospitals prepare a "drug formulary," which lists only a few hundred drugs that are regularly available in the hospital pharmacy.

With the freedom of hundreds of pharmaceutical companies to manufacture drugs and, formerly, the freedom to make grandiose claims about their benefits, there were bound to be abuses, which led sometimes to serious tragedies. As a result, the U.S. government has been stimulated to enact a sequence of "pure food and drug control" laws and regulations, which have greatly restricted the "freedom" of drug manufacturers. The requirements of these laws will be discussed later, but here it may simply be noted that the abuses existing in a very permissive health care system have given rise to legal constraints, for protection of the population, more sweeping than in more cooperative health care systems.

There has also been virtually complete freedom to establish pharmacies in the United States. As a result there are some 51,000 drugstores or one for every 4500 population—a ratio greatly in excess of needs. (Each drugstore normally has several pharmacists.) To survive economically, the average drugstore must sell many products outside of drugs. This may offer certain conveniences for people, but it means that much of the pharmacist's education is wasted, and other functions that might be performed by pharmacies, such as health education or certain routine screening tests, are not done.

Health Knowledge

Every health care system depends on knowledge about health and disease, and the application of knowledge through various technologies. A vast store of knowledge, of course, has been accumulated from the observations and experience of past centuries, but in the modern world new knowledge is increasingly acquired from scientific research.

Biomedical research is usually very costly, so that most of it is done in the economically affluent countries. In the very permissive setting of the U.S. health care system, research on countless medical problems is done at every medical school (about 125 institutions) and many other university departments or schools related to the health sciences. The topics to be investigated have customarily been determined by each scientist, according to his personal interests. In the early decades of the twentieth century, philanthropic bodies like the Rockefeller Foundation gave grants to universities for medical research and conducted such research itself (in the Rockefeller Institute). The federal government operated a relatively small Hygienic Laboratory for investigating selected problems of communicable disease. Most biomedical research, however, was done by medical faculty members, often in university-affiliated hospitals.

Since about 1940, these research policies have changed. In order to encourage research on problems of special public interest, the federal government has provided an increasing volume of research grants in selected fields. At the same time, national research institutes have been established for governmental work in these fields. The National Cancer Institute, for example, conducts research on a wide range of problems relevant to cancer and, in addition, makes hundreds of grants each year to investigators throughout the United States and even in other countries. Applications must be submitted for these grants, and they are reviewed by committees of scientists (appointed by the government) who evaluate them for support or rejection. No scientist is compelled to work on the cancer problem, but the availability of relatively large financing in this field obviously has an influence. In this way, government shapes medical research indirectly. A more direct strategy is the posing of certain specific research questions by government, with solicitation of proposals; many proposals—for example, on the relationship between coffee drinking and pancreatic cancer—may be submitted, but usually only one is chosen and finalized by a research contract.

Aside from government-funded research, conducted mainly (but not solely) by universities, pharmaceutical companies conduct a substantial amount of research on drugs and their effects on disease. These companies also give grants to medical scientists and clinicians, who are asked to investigate new products. Clinical research (i.e., on patients) must be carried out under strictly prescribed conditions, to protect the welfare of all "human subjects." With respect to sociomedical (as distinguished from biomedical) research, many governmental grants go to nonacademic firms devoted to health care management or administration.

SOURCES OF ECONOMIC SUPPORT

Most of the discussion of the organizational structure of health programs has explicitly or implicitly made reference to the sources of economic support. Governmental health programs are supported mainly by tax revenues, and voluntary agencies are supported mainly by charitable donations. Private market providers of health care, on the other hand, may be supported by complex combinations of payments by private families, tax revenues from one branch of government, social insurance from another branch, voluntary insurance, and still other sources. In this section, we will attempt to clarify the mixtures of different kinds of economic support found in the U.S. health care system.

Quantitative data on the various sources of economic support for a health care system, or on health expenditures, are not easily collected. It happens that in the United States, where problems of health economics have been debated for decades, such data are relatively abundant. These have been gathered both from household surveys and by soliciting information directly from major sources, such as voluntary insurance programs and government agencies.

In 1981, the U.S. population spent directly or indirectly about $275 billion on the health care system. This included expenditures for all components of the system discussed in this chapter, except the education of health manpower (in the U.S. "national accounts," these expenditures are included as part of the education sector). It included both recurrent and capital expenditures that year—recurrent ones, of course, being far greater than capital. This large outlay amounted to 9.6 percent of gross national product (GNP), a percentage which has been rising steadily for the last half-century.

The sources of these large health expenditures reflect a great deal about the sociopolitical characteristics of the U.S. health care system. The great bulk of them are for health services, accounting for 95.3 percent of the total (the balance of 4.7 percent being for medical research and construction of health facilities), and their distribution in 1980 was as follows:

Source	Percent
Personal individuals and families	28.5
Charitable donations	1.0
Management of enterprises	0.2
Voluntary health insurance	30.7
All private	(60.4)
Social insurance	14.4
Federal government revenues	14.2
State and local government revenues	11.0
All public	(39.6)
All sources	100.0

In very broad terms, it is evident that more than 60 percent of all U.S. health service expenditures come from private sources (or the private sector), and less than 40 percent come from all public or public sector sources. These relationships epitomize the permissiveness of the U.S. health care system and help to explain many aspects of its delivery patterns, to be discussed below. The trend, nevertheless, has been clearly toward a diminishing role for private household spending and an enlarging role for the major collective mechanisms: voluntary insurance, social insurance, and government revenues.

The seven sources of economic support listed above are actually very crude, and a proper clarification would require elaboration; space allows only a little. The "individuals and family" source refers to out-of-pocket expenditures, including repayment of personal loans, but does not include personal payment of insurance premiums. A large share of out-of-pocket expenditures goes to payment for ambulatory medical and dental care, and for drugs, which are not very well buffered by either voluntary or social insurance. Personal expenditures include the cost-sharing requirements under insurance (e.g., deductible amounts or co-payments), as well as the payment of charges not protected by insurance at all.

The very small percentage of funds derived from charitable donations may appear surprising, particularly insofar as it includes money spent by large philanthropic foundations (Rockefeller, Ford, Johnson, etc.) on health projects, as well as the donations of small sums to voluntary health agencies by millions of people. In absolute terms, the voluntary donations from charitable sources for health purposes have risen over the years, but the rise of expenditures from the other sources has been much greater—hence, the small percentage. The same applies basically to expenditures by the management of enterprises for the health protection of workers.

The source of funds identified as voluntary health insurance is composed of hundreds of separate organizations. Commercial insurance companies selling policies for health care number around one thousand, and nonprofit Blue Cross and Blue Shield plans paying for hospital and doctor's care number about 120. Other insurance organizations—variously characterized as "prepaid health plans" or "health maintenance organizations" or by other terms—amount to about another 500 entities. The great majority of people protected by these insurance programs are covered through their employment, and the premiums payable are typically shared between employee and employer—the latter usually paying the greater share or the entire amount. The percentages of persons covered by different types of insurance organization in the United States in 1982 were approximately as follows:

Commercial insurance companies	48
Blue Cross and Blue Shield	30
Prepaid health plans	10
None	12
All types of insurance	100

Social insurance in the U.S. health care system has three major components. One is the mandatory hospital insurance for the aged beneficiaries of the social security program. Second is the nonmandatory but governmental insurance for doctor's care and certain other medical services for the same population of elderly persons. Together these two are known as "Medicare," which is administered by the federal government, with the assistance of about 150 private "fiscal intermediaries" who make the direct payments to hospitals, doctors, and others. Much smaller in their total expenditures are the 50 state programs of "worker's compensation" for occupational injuries or illnesses; each of these is different, but a common feature is the payment of insurance premiums by employers. The expenditures relevant here are those made for medical purposes, and not for wage replacements.

General U.S. government revenues, as a source of health expenditures, include taxation levied at several political levels. The breakdown in 1980 was roughly 56 percent from federal government sources and 44 percent from state and local government sources. The major health function on which both federal and state revenues are spent is for medical care of the poor, principally through Medicaid. Federal taxation revenues are derived mainly from individual and corporate income taxes. State revenues come mainly from income and sales taxes. Local government revenues are derived mainly from taxes on property (real estate). The long-term trends have been toward an increase in the federal share of governmental health expenditures, although in recent years (under the Reagan administration) this trend has changed.

The health purposes for which the funds from these several sources are spent are very varied. Hospital care, for example, is supported predominantly by voluntary insurance and by social insurance; drugs and dental care are supported predominantly by individuals and families; public health activities (largely preventive) are supported predominantly by government revenues. Physician's care is supported by significant shares from all major sources of funding. The total matrix of economic sources and health purposes in the U.S. health care system is extremely complex, but the distribution of overall expenditures for

different health purposes (from all economic sources) in 1980 was as
follows:

Health Purpose	Percent of Expenditure
Hospital care (all types)	40.3
Skilled nursing home care	8.4
Physician's care (ambulatory and in-patient)	18.9
Dental care	6.4
Drugs and supplies	7.8
Other personal health care	6.3
Health care insurance administration	4.2
Public health services	3.0
Medical research	2.2
Health facility construction	2.5
All purposes	100.0

Trends in the above percentages have been toward devotion of increasing shares of the total expenditures to care in hospitals and nursing
homes. As a share of GNP, the total expenditures for health purposes
have also tended to rise.

MANAGEMENT OF THE SYSTEM

Just as financing is essential for the support of health care systems, so is
management. System management in this context is regarded as including four major activities: planning, administration, regulation, and
evaluation. Each of these activities is closely related to the others.
Problems of terminology, furthermore, may result in a certain action
being regarded as deliberate planning in one system, normal administration in a second system, and official regulation in a third. It will be
clearest, therefore, to consider all four of these aspects of management
together, as they are practiced in the health care system of the United
States.

In the permissive United States, all four aspects of management
stress local responsibility and private sponsorship. The role of government, in general, is kept to a minimum. In the U.S., planning for health
care or any other purpose was so long identified with Soviet communism

that it did not appear in any national health legislation until the end of World War II. In 1946, the national Hospital Survey and Construction Act (Hill-Burton) required that federal grants to the states for hospital construction be conditional on the preparation by the state of a "master plan," in which each hospital would theoretically have a designated role in a regionalized system. Not until 1967 did health planning go beyond this, to consider other resources and services, through a program of federal grants to some 200 local "comprehensive health planning" agencies. These bodies were mainly advisory, and in 1974, legislation was enacted to give local health planning agencies greater powers, particularly with respect to hospital construction. Very significantly, however, these local agencies were almost entirely nongovernmental, and very few of them had any connections with local departments of health.

The U.S. comprehensive health planning law of 1967 was passed as a sequel to the first national social insurance program for medical care of the aged (Medicare) and the large public medical care program for the poor (Medicaid). It would seem significant that the need for general health planning was not appreciated until a substantial amount of health money was to pass through government channels. With such public visibility of health expenditures, one can appreciate that there would be political concern that the funds be wisely spent—greater than such concern for purely private expenditures.

In a sense, any deliberate governmental or nongovernmental action, in which resources are to be allocated in some systematic way (outside the mechanisms of the free market), constitutes planning. In this sense, health planning in the United States and elsewhere can be traced to the establishment of the first hospital or the organization of the first department of public health. As customarily used, however, health planning applies to the actions of an agency which functions over and above the health resources and health organizations themselves, exerting an influence on their courses of action. In this sense, health planning in the United States has been very weak, indeed. Insofar as it has had any noticeable influence, it has been confined to the construction of hospitals, and the decisions have been made by agencies that are both local and nongovernmental. Insofar as the national government has played a part, it has been to issue "guidelines"—not regulations or official standards.

General health administration in the United States, like health planning, is characterized by decentralization and voluntarism. This goes beyond the constitutional requirements of state sovereignty. In the Medicare program, for example, the law might have authorized payments to health care providers through branch offices of the federal government; instead, payments are made to (and relationships maintained with) providers by numerous "fiscal intermediaries," which are not only local bodies but in every instance nongovernmental. Likewise, many federally authorized and financed health programs are implemented by grants to local agencies, below the level of the 50 state governments. There are about 3100 county governments and a much larger number of municipal governments, to which such health grants may be made, but a major share of them are voluntary nongovernmental bodies. This applies, for example, to grants for mental health services and grants for various types of community health centers. It also applies to federal grants for hospital construction or renovation.

To underscore the emphasis on local and nongovernmental decision making, almost all federally supported health programs must be governed or advised by a board of local citizens. Sometimes law requires that a majority of the governing board must be "consumers," rather than "providers" of health care. When some health program standard is issued at the state level, at the local level the standard may typically be applied with great leeway. The policies on the education of doctors and other health personnel are essentially up to each educational institution. Within the structure of state governments, the distribution of authority for health matters is so diverse that no two of the 50 states are exactly alike. Likewise within local governments, there is nearly always a "department of health," but the exact scope of activities carried out is hardly ever the same in two such departments of the same state or another state. Because of the multiplicity of health agencies at local and state levels, coordinating councils of various sorts abound—sometimes for health as a whole and sometimes in special fields, such as care of the aged or promotion of mental health.

Insofar as health administration may be characterized by its "style," it is mainly participatory rather than autocratic. Both in the private and the public sectors, rewards and advancement go to the supervisor who seeks everyone's opinion before reaching a decision. Meetings are held on every possible occasion to permit maximum discussion of problems. Though some of this democratic style of administration may be more apparent than real, there is no question about the theoretical preferences. National tradition in the U.S. opposes "bureaucracy" and glorifies "efficiency" and informality. In health program administration, this tends to mean delegation of great authority from higher to lower levels and relatively limited accountability through reporting back to the top. Yet information systems on health services rendered in a program are relatively well developed—to a great extent because such information serves as a basis for financial support.

Regulation in the U.S. health care system, somewhat paradoxically, is highly developed. To some extent, because of the easygoing form of administration just reviewed, many problems and abuses have developed; in response, regulations have been imposed to prevent further abuses. This is seen in the licensure of physicians which, prior to about 1870, was extremely loose and permissive; scores of poor-quality medical schools graduated physicians of very limited competence. As a result, the state governments developed their own examinations that had to be passed, over and above the academic examinations. Somewhat similar has been the development of regulatory legislation on drugs. In the nineteenth century, hundreds of uncontrolled pharmaceutical companies made extravagant and unjustified claims about their products. New drugs were put on the market, without proper testing of their safety (not to mention their efficacy), resulting in tragic deaths of patients. In response, drug control legislation, first enacted in 1906, has become progressively more rigorous.

With respect to specialization in medicine, regulation in the United States was initiated entirely outside of government. Starting with ophthalmology in 1916, "specialty board certification" was developed in one specialized medical or surgical discipline after another. Soon all the specialty boards came under the general jurisdiction of the nongovernmental American Medical Association—more than 50 fields, counting main specialties and subspecialties. Specific regimes of postgraduate training are required in each field, culminating in examinations. Although entirely private in its management, specialty board certification is recognized fully by government for purposes of reimbursement or eligibility to participate in certain public programs. Regarding basic medical licensure by the states, it is significant that the first action to simplify procedures, through a nationally uniform examination, was also taken by a nongovernmental body, the National Board of Medical Examiners.

Regulation by nongovernmental bodies has shown similar development in other fields. In the U.S. "open staff" hospital before 1920, each doctor was theoretically his own master, free to do almost anything he wished. As a consequence, some extremely poor medical and surgical work was done. In reaction, the hospital medical staffs, themselves, set up "bylaws" to govern what would be permitted within the hospital. In 1917, the American College of Surgeons, a private society, formulated standards for granting its approval of a hospital's policies (especially the medical staff procedures), and in 1952 the nongovernmental Joint Commission on Accreditation of Hospitals was organized. Similarly, professional associations established "codes of ethics." Health insurance organizations set their own rules and regulations. These were all outside the sphere of government, but their control over individual behavior could be just as great. Often such nongovernmental initiative has been taken deliberately to forestall governmental regulation. Sometimes a regulatory strategy may itself be abused, as in the case of professional ethics, which have been invoked to inhibit innovations in health care delivery.

Finally, the judicial system provides a certain type of regulation in the U.S. health care system. The patient who believes that a physician or hospital has brought him harm may bring suit in a court of law. The outcomes of such law suits are unpredictable (especially since they are usually tried by juries, and lawyers may be very skillful in their pleading), so that the great majority of cases are settled out of court. Whether settled or tried in court, law suits are a costly process, so that nearly all practicing physicians carry malpractice insurance, which has become increasingly expensive. Regardless of the merits of most malpractice claims, they have served to induce physicians and hospitals to discipline themselves—another form of self-regulatory response to the whole permissive character of the U.S. health care system.

Evaluation has also become highly developed in the U.S. health care system for reasons somewhat similar to those involving regulation. So much freedom has characterized the delivery of health services, and their costs have risen so rapidly, that many people were bound to raise questions about the quality and value of those services. When services became increasingly financed by government or by large groups of people, rather than by individuals, the questions became more insistent. As a response, various methods of evaluation have been developed in the U.S. health services. "Medical audits" have been promoted in hospitals, based on reviews of patient records in relation to explicit or implicit quality criteria. Under the national Medicare and Medicaid laws, there are requirements for qualitative "peer reviews" in every community. Most voluntary health insurance organizations also have developed surveillance procedures to detect cases of improper or unjustified medical service. The line between quality control and cost control is not sharp, but it is clear that the U.S. health care system has generated many forms of evaluation in pursuit of both objectives.

DELIVERY OF HEALTH SERVICES

The several major components of health care systems we have reviewed culminate in the encounter between a provider and a recipient of health service. To distinguish this more personal process from the other components of the system, it is customarily called the "delivery of health services." These services may be analyzed as primary, secondary, and tertiary, plus a fourth category, in which all levels of service are directed toward selected populations or selected disorders.

Primary Health Services

Primary health services include a wide range of preventive measures plus first-encounter medical care of the patient with a health care provider—usually a doctor in the industrialized countries. Preventive measures may be environmental (e.g., water purification), educational, or personal, but here we will consider only personal prevention. Common forms of personal preventive measures are immunizations, surveillance of expectant mothers and babies, and adult examinations for detection of chronic diseases.

In the United States primary health service is delivered predominantly by private physicians in their private offices. Increasing proportions of doctors, however, are joining together in small medical groups or group practices (three or more doctors working together and sharing their income in some way), particularly doctors in various specialties. In 1980, nevertheless, the majority were still in individual practice. The patient ordinarily pays for this service out of pocket; even though most of the population has some health insurance protection, it usually does not pay for ambulatory primary care. In fact, even if there is third-party payment for ambulatory services, as under Medicare, preventive services are specifically excluded. Hence, most immunizations are given by private pediatricians, most prenatal examinations by private obstetricians, and general medical check-ups by private internists.

There are, indeed, organized public health clinics for these personal preventive services, but they tend to serve only 15–20 percent of the population, mainly the poor. Children are sometimes immunized in schools, and industrial workers may get routine medical examinations in larger size plants. Multiple screening tests may be done at work places or elsewhere, and the patient with any positive finding is typically referred to a private physician.

The treatment aspects of primary health service are also most often rendered in private medical offices, typically those of specialists; general practitioners or family practice specialists constitute only a small fraction of the doctors. Patients of low income, however, frequently seek primary medical care in the outpatient department of hospitals, most often in the "emergency room." Scheduled clinics in various specialties are held only in a small proportion of hospitals, usually in large cities. Since about 1965, various types of community health centers have been established in poverty sections of large cities and some rural areas. At these units, a wide range of primary services are offered by salaried doctors and allied staffs; only a small fraction of overall ambulatory care encounters, however, occur in these settings.

Secondary and Tertiary Health Services

A high development of secondary and tertiary health services is particularly characteristic of the United States, with its very permissive health care system. Until relatively recent times, any community or group that could raise the money to build a hospital was free to do so, and to furnish the facility with whatever sophisticated diagnostic or treatment equipment it could afford. The same freedom applied to physicians, who could specialize in whatever field for which they could find postgraduate training, so that more than 85 percent of physicians became specialists. An approach to regionalization of hospital facilities was made in 1946, with the Hospital Survey and Construction Act, and again in 1966, with the Act for Regional Medical Programs on Heart Disease, Cancer and Stroke, but the regionalization concept remains largely a theoretical idea. In reality, almost any patient is free to consult any high-powered specialist for a minor problem (provided he can pay the cost), and almost any doctor is free to hospitalize his private patient for diagnosis and treatment, even if they could well be given in the office of a general practitioner.

The concept of a pyramidal framework of health service, in which the patient is seen by primary care personnel before having access to secondary or tertiary care, is implemented in certain "health maintenance organizations" (HMOs) in the United States. HMOs, however, cover only about 10 percent of the population. The free-wheeling pattern noted above characterizes health care delivery in the average community. Patients have direct access to specialists in private practice, and only a minority of the average specialist's patients come on referral from another doctor. In general hospitals, medical staff organization is typically "open," so that almost any qualified physician applying for staff affiliation is granted it. A general hospital of 100 beds in a city might have 100 physicians and surgeons on its medical staff, although only 10 or 20 of them might have patients hospitalized at any one time. Each doctor is responsible for his own patients, and seeking consultation from another staff member is entirely up to him. Because of this great permissiveness, and the hazards of improper care, the medical staffs of most American hospitals have established numerous self-disciplinary committees—on surgery, drug therapy, length of stay of patients, record-keeping, and so on—to monitor each other.

Most general hospital patients in the United States are protected by voluntary insurance, and hospitals have customarily been paid their charges for each case. Insurance also typically pays the doctor his private fees for inpatient service. Nevertheless, a slowly increasing proportion of hospital doctors have become based in the hospital full time and paid by salary. This has long applied to pathologists and radiologists, but it is becoming more frequent for internists, surgeons, and other specialists who serve as the full-time heads of clinical departments and as heads of outpatient services, of continuing medical education, of medical rehabilitation, and other fields. There are also some HMO hospitals with entirely full-time salaried medical staffs, similar to those in governmental general hospitals, like the network of the Veterans Administration. Government legislation in the 1980s is also leading to a shift in the methods of paying for hospital services, from retrospective charges to prospective rates based on the diagnostic category (the diagnosis-related group or DRG) of each case. In spite of these trends, as of the early 1980s the "open staff" general hospital was the norm in America; only for mental hospitals, some special government general hospitals, and institutions attached to medical schools is the full-time salaried "closed staff" of physicians the usual pattern.

Finally, in the United States the large urban public hospital, limited essentially to serving the poor, is an important component of the pattern of delivery for secondary and tertiary care. It is a hangover of the late nineteenth and early twentieth centuries, when programs such as Medicaid were not available to finance care of the poor in the customary community hospital. With such financial support programs in the "mainstream" hospital system, these special public hospitals now serve principally low-income patients not eligible for Medicaid or other third-party support. Because of rising costs of hospital maintenance and restrictions in local revenues (on which most of these hospitals depend), public hospitals for the poor face chronic financial difficulties.

Care of Special Populations and Disorders

In all types of health care system, there are special programs—encompassing primary, secondary, and tertiary care—for the care of certain population groups, and for the control of certain disorders. For various historical and political reasons, as well as for economy and efficiency, special forms of delivery of health care have been developed for these populations and disorders.

In the United States health care system, where private buying and selling of health service is the norm, it is noteworthy that—as in virtually all countries—military personnel are served by a highly structured and comprehensive health care program, financed entirely by government funds. The Army, Navy, Air Force, and Marines each has its own network of health facilities—hospitals, clinics, and field posts. All personnel are public employees, salaried according to their military ranks (without relation to the specific services they render). The same basic structure prevails in times of war or peace. Health promotion and prevention are emphasized and integrated with the delivery of treatment services. Even after retirement, high-ranking officers continue to be entitled to these comprehensive services, without personal costs. If service of a highly specialized type is needed, but available only at a distant place, the patient will be transported there promptly; if this resource is private, the bill is paid by the military establishment.

After military service, the U.S. veteran becomes entitled to a remarkably broad range of medical care. If a disorder is connected with military service, its care is a responsibility of the federal Veterans Administration for life. For any other disorder suffered by the veteran, hospital care is provided through a nationwide network of VA facilities (usually affiliated with medical schools to assure high quality), so long as the veteran states it would cause him financial "hardship" to obtain the care privately. Normally, about 75 percent of VA hospital beds are occupied by veterans with such conditions, unrelated to military service. The United States is unique in supporting so broad a scope of health services for veterans—a fact doubtless related to the lack of a national health insurance program for the general population. After World War I, the political demands of veterans for such special benefits led to public action.

Another specially favored population in the United States is the American Indians, who are provided a comprehensive range of services through special clinics and hospitals in or near Indian reservations throughout the nation. For years these public services were managed by the Bureau of Indian Affairs of the Department of Interior, but in the 1950s they were transferred to the administration of the U.S. Public Health Service.

Other programs for the health care of special populations in the United States include those for railroad workers, for employees of special projects such as the Tennessee Valley Authority, or for migratory farm workers. Merchant seamen are another population for whom a special network of federal hospitals has long been operated at major port cities. Special programs for industrial workers and schoolchildren have been already noted, and in colleges and universities the scope of health services for students is typically comprehensive. In contrast to customary U.S. patterns of health care delivery, through private medical and allied practitioners, services in all these programs are provided by salaried personnel working in organized frameworks.

Among disorders for which special subsystems of health care delivery are organized in the United States, mental illness is probably most important. A large share of ambulatory psychiatric care is, indeed, provided by individual psychiatrists in the mainstream of private medical practice, but a substantial amount of such care is furnished to low-income patients through thousands of special mental health clinics, under public or voluntary auspices. These clinics are staffed typically by teams of psychiatrists, psychologists, social workers, nurses, and others—all working on a salary basis. Hospitalization for mental illness is predominantly in special mental hospitals, financed and operated by state governments (although general hospitals have been increasingly admitting short-term patients with psychiatric diagnoses). Tuberculosis, before its steep decline in incidence and prevalence, also warranted a special network of clinics and hospitals (sanitaria) for its detection and care.

LOOKING AHEAD

The highly permissive and pluralistic character of the U.S. health care system implies the type of problems encountered. Although viewpoints will inevitably vary among different observers, there is a broad consensus that health care costs have been rising excessively and much too rapidly. The free market in medical care has been so uncontrolled, even for services paid for by governmental insurance, that prices have spiraled to much higher levels than the general consumer price index. The Medicare program for medical care for the aged, for example, permits the doctor (by not "accepting assignment") to charge the patient any fee he wishes. Hospital charges have been mounting to especially towering heights, as hospital technology has increased, as hospital personnel per patient have multiplied, and as salaries have risen.

With the escalation of costs, access of the lower income groups to needed care has become more difficult. Government programs to finance care for the poor, like Medicaid, have been cut back at both the federal and state levels. Even in the social insurance Medicare program, co-payments required from the patient have increased, so that the heavy burden of illness in the aged is getting attention only with increasing difficulty. The whole political environment created by the Reagan Administration in the 1980s has promoted reduction in public expenditures for all human services and much greater reliance on private sector financing.

A special aspect of this ideology has been a striking privatization of the health care system. More and more voluntary nonprofit hospitals have been bought out by commercial hospital chains. Voluntary and even public hospitals have been turned over to management by private corporations, in the expectation that this will enhance efficiency and productivity. Up to this writing, evidence of such effects has not been shown, and some studies have even shown higher costs associated with commercialization of hospital service.

To stem the tide of rising medical and hospital costs, major reliance has been on promoting competition among providers. The "preferred provider organization" (PPO) has been spawned as a mechanism by which groups of doctors and/or hospitals agree to serve certain public or private beneficiaries at competitively lower prices. For some years the prepaid health maintenance organization (HMO) has shown the economies achievable by modification of physician incentives, especially in hospital use, and now a number of variations on the HMO theme are being explored. Although competition is politically favored in preference to regulation, the very largest innovation in public medical care policy has been essentially regulatory. This has been, as noted earlier, the introduction of prospective payment to hospitals according to the "diagnosis-related group" (DRG) of each patient under Medicare (and in some states for all insurance payers), rather than by charges retrospectively for each unit of service.

While the pressure of rising costs has been responsible for many of the changes being seen in the U.S. health care system, long-term forces with broader objectives than cost containment continue their impacts. The whole movement for social financing of health care, to assure its availability to everyone, continues. Legislation for national health insurance lost the priority position it held in the 1970s, but there can be no doubt that it will move forward again. Hawaii enacted mandatory state health insurance in 1975, and other states may follow suit, along the lines that led to national legislation in Canada. So much depends, of course, on the character of the political party elected to national power in 1988.

The enthusiastic promotion of prevention and sound lifestyle, which has come to occupy center stage in recent years, is bound to continue. To expect this policy to result in lesser need for medical care, however, is an idle wish. As men and women live longer, due to the prevention or postponement of both communicable and noncommunicable disease, they live on to the age when cancer or other disorders strike. Moreover, they live on with diseases under control, with hypertension, diabetes, glaucoma, arthritis, cardiovascular problems, and other disorders that are not cured but are controlled by good medical care. Maintenance of the quality of life in the company of chronic disease is quite possible, but it has its costs.

Continuing specialization and technological advances render the solo medical practitioner more obsolete each day. Despite the glories in America of individual freedom, the grouping of doctors, nurses, technicians, and others in teams—either under public or private auspices—is doubtless the wave of the future. Organization of health care delivery means that fee-for-service payments will be replaced by various social mechanisms of financing and all personnel, including doctors, will eventually be paid salaries, based on their qualifications, responsibilities, and hours of work. The perverse incentives of fees-per-medical-act will be replaced by incentives to win the respect of one's peers.

All this means more deliberate planning of the U.S. health care system, more rational regulation to promote quality and avert abuse, and more strategies that will help assure the health services that each person needs. The World Health Organization goal of Health For All by the Year 2000 should certainly be attainable in the United States. The heterogeneity and pluralism of the U.S. health culture will certainly not vanish, but organization and coordination will enable it to achieve harmonious performance and equity in the years ahead.

Chapter **2**

The Advancing Organization of Ambulatory Care*

Assaults by the Reagan Administration on long-established U.S. health policies have been distressing to millions of Americans. After half a century of progress in improving the distribution of health services to the population, a sudden reversal is upon us. Many health workers have become pessimistic about ever achieving an equitable health care system in the United States.

Yet if one looks around the world at other industrialized nations and considers how their health care systems have evolved, one can see current events in better perspective. As in so many other countries, and indeed as in America's own past, there are rises and falls in all movements toward social goals. We are now in a downward slope of the trend line, but there is every reason to believe that the direction will change before long. In this belief, one may expect that long-term trends toward more effective organization of all types of health services will continue. An increasingly important component of the health services is ambulatory care, on which this chapter is focused. The prospect of enhanced organization for the delivery of such care has many implications for health personnel.

---

*For citations and great detail on the subject of this article, please see M. I. Roemer, *Ambulatory Health Services in America: Past, Present, and Future* (Rockville, Md.: Aspen Systems Corp., 1981).

HISTORICAL BACKGROUND

Personal health care has long been provided to patients in four principal settings: a patient's home, a practitioner's office, a hospital (or other bed facility), or an ambulatory care clinic of some type. Over the last century, however, the mix of these settings has changed strikingly, and this has created increasing demands for nurses and many types of allied health personnel.

A century ago, in 1880, medical care for most people in America was divided essentially between the doctor's office and the patient's home. Hospitals were few and were devoted largely to giving care to the very poor and to patients with extremely serious illnesses. Organized clinics were also rare, limited largely to "dispensaries" for the poor in big cities.

Over the next few decades, hospitals were built everywhere in America. In 1873 there were only 178 hospitals in the nation, many of which were solely for the mentally ill. By 1910, general hospitals had been established in almost every community, and a count of them by the American Medical Association came to nearly 4400.

After about 1920, as transportation improved by both common carriers and family automobiles, patients could be much more mobile. Demands for medical care were rising and doctors became busier. Increasingly, they expected patients to come to their offices. Home calls decreased steadily, so that they account today for hardly 1.0 percent of the patient–doctor encounters in the United States.

For many reasons discussed below, clinics for organized provision of ambulatory care came to be developed under several different sponsorships. The two decades 1900–1920 were a period of rapid growth for public health departments and voluntary health agencies. Special clinics for babies or for tackling certain diseases were major components of their programs. Stimulated by worker's compensation laws, industries began to engage nurses and doctors. To be on guard against communicable diseases, schools set up clinics staffed by nurses and part-time doctors. After World War I, many physicians began to join together in private group practice clinics, and these grew with greater momentum after World War II.

In the 1960s, America seemed to rediscover poverty, and among many responses was the development by the U.S. Office of Economic Opportunity (OEO) of "neighborhood health centers" for general ambulatory medical care. Located mainly in urban slum areas, these modern-day dispensaries were established under several different auspices. The old dispensaries had long been replaced almost everywhere by hospital outpatient departments (OPDs). Various public agencies beyond the OEO supported the development of community health centers that offered a wide range of treatment and preventive services. Clinics for selected beneficiaries—military personnel, veterans, merchant seamen, American Indians, and so on—had also long been operated by the federal government.

Another sponsorship of ambulatory care clinics was encouraged in the 1970s, called "health maintenance organizations" or HMOs. These involved essentially the linkage of an organized group of doctors and other health personnel with an insurance plan that financed a broad range of services. Such arrangements, formerly called "prepaid group medical practices," had been evolving as a nonorthodox pattern of health care in America, but now it became "respectable" and was promoted by federal government subsidies.

Thus, by 1980 one could identify in the United States some eight different types of organized ambulatory health care, generally known as "clinics." Based on their *sponsorships,* these were as follows:

1. Hospital outpatient departments
2. Public health agency clinics
3. Industrial health service units
4. School health clinics
5. Voluntary agency clinics
6. Private group medical practices
7. Health centers or clinics of other public agencies
8. Health maintenance organizations

The numbers of these clinics have all increased almost steadily over the last 50 years, and the range of health services they provide has broadened. The same would tend to be true if one were to classify clinics by their *objectives,* such as being for mental health purposes, for cancer detection, for children, for rural people, for the urban poor, or for emergency care. This variety of arrangements for the organized delivery of ambulatory health care, as we shall see, is slowly replacing the individual doctor's office as the setting in which people receive medical services in the United States.

Clinics of all types, of course, mean that organized teams of health personnel are at work. The extent of staffing and organization naturally varies among the eight types of clinic and also within each type. In general, however, health teams require various categories of allied health personnel beyond the physician. A few words about each type of clinic and its personnel implications in modern America may be of interest.

HOSPITAL OUTPATIENT DEPARTMENTS (OPDS)

Hospital OPDs offer three general types of ambulatory service: emergency care, scheduled specialist services, and referral services. Most familiar to people is the "emergency room," where patients may come at any hour of the day or night for medical help. About 80 percent of the nation's 7100 hospitals offer these services, and the volume of patient visits has been steadily increasing. In reality, most visits to emergency rooms are for conditions that are not really "urgent" from a medical viewpoint, although they may be distressing for the patient. Patients of any income level may seek emergency OPD service, although the principal users tend to be low-income persons who do not have immediate access to physicians.

Scheduled OPD clinics are typically classified by medical specialties—surgery, pediatrics, gynecology—and they are held at specified times each week. Ordinarily they are restricted to the poor and are found in about 30 percent of hospitals. Referred OPD services—typically diagnostic procedures—are services for private patients sent to the hospital by doctors who lack appropriate equipment or personnel in their offices. Almost every general hospital provides such services for the patients of physicians on their medical staffs.

All three types of OPD clinics depend for their operation on a variety of trained health personnel. Hospital nurses are usually essential, and in larger facilities they may be assigned full time to the OPD. Clinics at all hospitals, of course, have the advantage of convenient access to other hospital resources, such as the laboratory, the x-ray department, electrocardiography, the pharmacy, and so on. Personnel in these several hospital departments, therefore, are serving outpatients as well as inpatients. Furthermore, in very large hospitals, laboratory, x-ray, and pharmaceutical personnel may be permanently attached to the OPD.

Scheduled clinics also often provide social workers to help patients cope with their problems of living.

PUBLIC HEALTH AGENCY CLINICS

Health departments or public health agencies conduct a variety of special clinics, oriented mainly to the prevention of disease. Important among these are clinics for tuberculosis control (often giving treatment as well as case-detection service), for child health (where immunizations, examinations, and education on child-rearing are provided), for prenatal care, for venereal disease (VD) control, and for mental health and other problems. In recent years, public health agencies have broadened the scope of their clinics to include family planning service (birth control), chronic disease detection, and also the general primary care of families.

Public health nurses are the mainstay of these clinics, in addition to part-time physicians who are mainly in private practice. Other personnel in public health clinics include health educators, nutritionists or dietitians, VD investigators, and various clerks. Mental health clinics typically have psychologists and social workers as well as psychiatrists on their staffs.

Health departments have sometimes been regarded in recent years as declining in importance. In fact, they have been expanding in number and scope, although the growth of other types of health agency has been more conspicuous. There are about two thousand local public health units in the nation, and, of course, a state health department exists in each of the 50 states. Beyond the personnel working in various clinics, public health agencies require sanitarians (to monitor environmental conditions), statisticians, health educators with specialized skills, and sometimes persons trained specifically in family planning.

INDUSTRIAL HEALTH SERVICE UNITS

The exact number of "in-plant" health units in the United States is not known, but there must be many thousands. Their degree of development varies greatly according to plant size, as measured by the number of employees. In small plants (with fewer than one hundred workers), health services are ordinarily quite rudimentary—often limited to a first-aid box and arrangements with some community health facility to which injured workers may be sent.

Very large plants (with more than 2500 workers) usually have some systematic in-plant health service, most often staffed by trained industrial nurses and part-time or full-time physicians. Industries vary greatly in the extent of their health hazards—mostly trauma (accidents) but also occupational diseases (such as silicosis, asbestosis, or lead poisoning). In white-collar firms, such as department stores or insurance companies, clinic services are mainly for minor, nonoccupational conditions. In a relatively small number of large firms, in-plant health services may be extended to provide employees with complete medical care for all disorders, whether or not job connected.

When an industry has special hazards because of toxic substances or harmful dust, industrial hygienists may be engaged periodically or permanently. These are personnel with special knowledge of factory or mining problems and methods by which they may be controlled. Industrial nurses and physicians, of course, can be better prepared for their work through special training programs. The federal Occupational Safety and Health Act of 1970 was a landmark in this field, even though there have been serious limitations in the implementation of regulations under it.

Long-term trends in American industry are toward the greater concentration of production in relatively fewer large corporations. While this tendency doubtless leads to many economic and social problems in the nation, it actually enhances the prospects of occupational health programs. These are typically organized and financed by management, and the costs are more easily borne in large establishments.

SCHOOL HEALTH CLINICS

There are about 60 million students in all school levels in the nation—primary, secondary, and universities or colleges. School facilities number about 110,000 (public and private), in almost all of which some type of organized, ambulatory health service is provided. Most often, the key health person is a part-time or full-time school nurse, usually engaged by the local education authorities but sometimes assigned by the public health agency. School physicians, who examine children to detect physical or mental disorders, are principally part-time private practitioners; in some large school districts, such as New York or Los Angeles, they may be full-time salaried doctors.

Childhood problems that may retard learning are naturally of greatest concern in school systems, so that special personnel beyond nurses and doctors are often appointed. There may be psychologists for identifying mental and emotional difficulties and occasionally medical social workers and special education teachers. For discovery of hearing defects (which may often be overlooked), audiologists are sometimes engaged to test the hearing of every child. Dental hygienists may also work in school systems to inspect teeth and to educate children about sound dental habits. At the university level, especially at campuses where the students are far from their family homes, comprehensive health programs, including both ambulatory care and hospitalization, are often provided.

VOLUNTARY AGENCY CLINICS

Voluntary health agencies focusing on special disorders—tuberculosis, cancer, heart disease, poliomyelitis, and so on—have operated in the United States for many years. Most of these are national associations with numerous local branches. Many of these societies, focusing on specific diseases, originated with the sponsorship of clinics. Their principal current activities stress the support of medical research and professional education; some voluntary agencies, however, still operate clinics, such as those for cancer detection sponsored by the American Cancer Society.

In addition to physicians and nurses, voluntary health agencies engage other types of personnel. Physical therapists play an important role in programs for crippled children and for patients with multiple sclerosis or other neurological disorders. Associations for the blind require personnel who can teach Braille reading, and agencies for the deaf may need teachers of sign language.

In the 1960s, a new type of nongovernmental clinic was started in many large American cities—the "free clinic." These units were usually initiated by youth groups with strong anti-Establishment attitudes. They chose not to use hospital OPDs or public health clinics, which they regarded as too bureaucratic. Instead, the young people would raise money for renting an empty store and purchasing drugs, while professional services were solicited and obtained on a voluntary basis from doctors, nurses, pharmacists, and others. For a time, some free clinics even came to be subsidized by local governments.

Usually the only staff member paid by a free clinic was the administrator or director, who had to be on duty at all times. Occasionally young men or women trained in health care administration would do this work. In recent years, many of the free clinics have closed down, but some have become sponsored by established agencies, including medical schools. Other similar "self-help" clinics are sponsored by feminist groups or groups devoted to holistic medicine.

PRIVATE GROUP MEDICAL PRACTICES

The medical profession itself is mainly responsible for the organization of group medical practices throughout the United States. In 1975 there were more than 7700 group practices—as defined by the American Medical Association: three or more physicians working together and sharing their earnings in some way. There are great variations in the size of group practices, but with 60,000 participating physicians, the average has 7.8 medical members. Multispecialty groups tend to be larger than those confined to a single specialty (such as surgery or radiology).

A major advantage of group medical practice is its capability to engage allied health personnel to an extent that would not be feasible for the solo practitioner. In 1975, there were 2.53 allied health workers for each doctor in group practice. Aside from nurses and clerical personnel found in every group practice, most also engage laboratory and x-ray technicians. A small percentage of medical groups engages health educators, dietitians, psychologists, pharmacists, social workers, dentists, and even podiatrists.

Group medical practice is growing very rapidly in the United States—probably more than any other type of organized ambulatory care. With teams of personnel, group practices tend to have higher productivity per physician-hour, although some economists have questioned this. In any case, it is clear that for the same medical workweek (about 50 hours), group practice physicians have higher net earnings than individual practitioners. If the current growth rate of grouping continues, it will soon become the predominant pattern of medical practice in the United States.

CLINICS OF OTHER PUBLIC AGENCIES

The numerous general clinics for certain federal beneficiaries have operated for many years—those for merchant seamen going back to 1798. Comprehensive "community health centers," supported by government and serving all low-income people in an area, have developed in the last two decades. Most of these health centers receive financial support from several different agencies, each of which issues reports on the number of facilities it helps. Because of this overlapping, it is difficult to derive an unduplicated count, but a careful estimate suggests that there are about one thousand such centers in the nation. (With recent federal cutbacks in health care budgeting, many of these will probably close down.)

Some of the rural health centers are modestly staffed, with only a single "nurse practitioner" in periodic contact with a physician. In the community health centers located in poverty districts of large cities, the staffing tends to be quite abundant. There may be physicians of several specialties, registered nurses, vocational nurses, laboratory technicians, health educators, physical therapists, psychologists, dental hygienists, pharmacists, records clerks, and others. Diverse patterns of organization and teamwork are followed.

For mental illness, various public ambulatory care programs have been organized. Independent psychiatric clinics, not attached to a hospital or other facility, have been operated for years by special governmental agencies (often departments of mental health). Since 1963 a national network of community mental health centers (CMHCs) has been developed. By 1979, there were seven hundred CMHCs, each offering a wide range of mental health services for both adults and children. Although locally sponsored by either public or private organizations, all were launched with government grants. Other public clinics address the problems of alcoholism and drug abuse.

The personnel requirements of facilities for ambulatory mental health services include psychologists, psychiatric social workers, psychiatrically trained nurses, carefully chosen receptionists, in addition to psychiatrists. Community outreach workers are a new type of personnel trained in recent years by ambulatory care programs, both general and mental. These are typically (but not always) young women from the neighborhood who may have no background in the health field but who understand local attitudes. After brief training, they visit families and encourage them to make use of the health services being offered.

HEALTH MAINTENANCE ORGANIZATIONS (HMOs)

A comprehensive scope of health services, both ambulatory and institutional, combined with annually fixed financial support by insurance are the main attributes of health maintenance organizations (HMOs). With federal subsidies through the 1970s, programs meeting the general definition of HMOs grew to more than two hundred in the nation, although by 1980 only about half had become "federally qualified." Their total membership of less than 9 million was only a small fraction of the national population, but their significance as a strategy for changing the pattern of health care delivery in this country has been increasingly appreciated.

Clinics in HMOs are staffed with virtually every type of health personnel. With the fiscal incentive of maximizing ambulatory care and keeping prudent restraints on the use of hospitals, the relative need for allied health personnel is great. They are required for laboratory work, rehabilitative therapy, drug dispensing, record-keeping, and other assignments. In addition, HMOs have special needs for administrative personnel to manage and oversee the entire program. Health care administrators, with various levels of qualification, must provide effective management for the enrollment of members, the recruitment of providers, and the control of the whole financial process supporting the program. Administration of HMOs is so complex that several university schools of public health and graduate schools of administration (business or public) offer special courses for training in this field.

CONCLUSION

This review of eight major types of organized ambulatory health care in America may clarify the wide range of personnel required for these programs. There are great difficulties in quantifying the overall national magnitude of organized ambulatory care, in contrast to service from individual medical practitioners. The numbers of patients visiting hospital OPDs, for example, or child health clinics of public health agencies are systematically reported each year, but for most types of clinic service one can only make the best possible estimates. The overall volume of patient–doctor encounters in the United States, in both individual and organized settings, is reported periodically by the U.S. National Center for Health Statistics (based on its continuing "Health Interview Survey"). In recent years this has amounted to about 5.0 visits per person per year, or somewhat more than one billion contacts for the U.S. national civilian population.

My own calculations from the best sources available show that in the mid-1970s about 50 percent of the ambulatory doctor–patient contacts in the United States took place in organized settings. All the evidence suggests that this proportion is steadily increasing. In another decade or two, it is quite likely that services from private solo medical practitioners in America will be exceptional. The organizing trends that have long characterized hospital care are coming now to characterize ambulatory care.

For allied health personnel, the implications of this trend are quite clear. The organization of functions in the health care system is not altogether different from that in other systems. Although the output of good health service requires far more humanistic sensitivities than the manufacture of hammers or screwdrivers, the processes are similar in certain respects. Greater efficiency in both activities can be achieved by the division of labor among different personnel and coordination of their work. With effective coordination and administration, a "product" of higher quality can be turned out at a relatively lower net cost. The administrative process itself creates other problems, but countless experiences in society have shown that they can be solved.

As noted earlier, health care administration demands skilled personnel at several levels. The graduate training of administrators in this field has come to be offered by dozens of universities; the curricula today are far richer and more diversified than those in the first schools of public health launched in the early part of this century. For middle management positions, undergraduate university courses have also been developed, including programs for preparing health record librarians, statisticians, accountants, and others.

A final aspect of organized ambulatory health care must be appreciated—its dependence on adequate economic support. The traditional method of paying for a doctor's care has been personal out-of-pocket spending; a fee is paid for each discrete service. With the advancing potentialities of biomedical science and the mounting costs of medical care, all sorts of collective or social methods of financing have been developed, indicating government revenues of various types, charitable donations, voluntary or mandatory insurance, and so on. Private medical practice, however, has been so firmly established in the United States and many other industrialized countries that even when financing has been collectivized, individual practitioners are still usually paid on the basis of a fee for each unit of service.

In organized ambulatory care, doctors, along with other personnel, are ordinarily paid not for each specific service but for the value of their time—hence payment by full- or part-time salaries. The sources of financial support for most types of clinics, moreover, are socially organized. Governmental tax support has become increasingly important. In the United States, governmental financing for all types of health service was about 14 percent of the total in 1930, and it has risen to more than 40 percent today. Another 30 percent of health care financing in the United States comes from voluntary insurance.

These social methods of economic support have obviously extended the availability of health care to more people. Both the quantity and quality of health services have risen. At the same time, the operation of organized health programs—including the ambulatory care discussed here—has become especially dependent on government. Changes in the political ideology of government can therefore have a great impact on the health care system.

Today the dominant viewpoint in the government of the United States favors a reversal of the trend in public financing that has prevailed over the last 50 years. Tax support for military purposes is being increased, while that for health and human services is being decreased. The private sector of the economy is being encouraged to assume responsibilities that have long been sustained in the public sector. The social forces behind the previous trends in health care have not disappeared, however. Motivated by objectives for attaining both equity and efficiency, they will surely continue to influence the contours of the American health care system. There is good reason to expect that, although the movement toward greater organization of both financing and delivery of health services may change direction for a while, in the long run it will continue forward.

Chapter **3**

The Development of Public Health in the United States

The position of public health agencies in the overall health sector of the United States has been determined by two major influences. One has been the capabilities within the field of public health—a field that may be defined as a population-based approach to promoting health, in contrast to the orientation of clinical medicine to treatment of individual patients. The second influence has been the external circumstances surrounding public health agencies in society, particularly the distribution of authority and responsibility in the health sector as a whole.

Both of these influences have changed over the years, resulting in differing positions for public health organization in various historical periods. The role of public health agencies can be best understood, therefore, by examining the health scene in the United States in the following periods of time:

Beginnings	1800–1870
Maturation in government	1870–1910
Focus on prevention	1910–1935
Expansion and development	1935–1960
Health care progress elsewhere	1960–1980

49

BEGINNINGS, 1800–1870

Public health activity arose in the United States in the first years of the nineteenth century. As in Europe, it first occurred in the largest cities in which concentrations of population led to the spread of communicable diseases. Typically, in response to epidemics, a board or commission would be appointed to make regulations for the maintenance of a sanitary environment. Even before microorganisms were recognized as causative agents of disease, the hazards of a dirty environment and contaminated water were recognized. John Snow in London had attributed a cholera epidemic to drinking polluted water drawn from the Thames River in 1849, long before the bacteria causing this disease had been described.

In New York City an epidemic of yellow fever occurred in 1798. A Board of Health, composed of leading citizens, had been established some years before to recommend measures for elimination of filth from the streets, for drainage of swamps, and other objectives of environmental sanitation. In 1804, a full-time city inspector of health was appointed. He and his staff were lodged in the New York Police Department, since the *enforcement* of sanitary regulations was seen as the central task. These personnel were not transferred to a separate agency under a permanent Board of Health until 1838. Similar developments occurred in Boston, Philadelphia, and a few other cities in this period.

The boards of health were concerned principally with the maintenance of a sanitary environment. Quarantine and isolation of patients with communicable diseases were also practiced, since contagiousness was realized (also before the identification of bacteria). Until the Civil War, boards of health were limited to large cities. In 1849, however, a Sanitary Commission was appointed in Massachusetts to survey health and sanitation problems in the whole state. The report of this commission, chaired by Lemuel Shattuck, appeared in 1850 and made recommendations on vital statistics (including the notification of communicable diseases), smallpox vaccination, many aspects of environmental sanitation, and health education of the general population on hygiene. To implement these ideas, the commission proposed a board of health with permanent staffing at the state level, along with similar boards in the government of every town. Not until after the Civil War—1869— however, was the first *state* board of health set up in Massachusetts.

PUBLIC HEALTH MATURATION IN GOVERNMENT, 1870–1910

As the United States settled down after the Civil War, a more firm structure of government gradually took shape in the main cities and in state capitals. With heavy immigration from Europe and the development of industry, cities grew rapidly as did problems of environmental sanitation. By the end of the nineteenth century, boards of health had been established within the governments of most large cities as well as at the state level.

In 1878, a National Quarantine Act was passed by Congress for the purpose of preventing the entry, by ships from Europe, of persons with communicable diseases. The surgeon general of the Marine Hospital Service (which had originated in 1798) was put in charge of quarantine procedures at the principal ports of the United States. In the next year, 1879, a National Board of Health was established by law for "foreign and interstate quarantine." By then, however, the sovereignty of the states on public health matters and other domestic affairs was well established; a National Board of Health was ahead of its time, and in 1883 Congress let it die through withholding appropriations.

Although boards of health and permanently staffed health departments under them were widespread features of state and local governments by 1900, their functions remained limited to the enforcement of sanitary regulations and of certain measures for the control of acute communicable disease. It was about 1860–1870 that the work of Louis Pasteur and others in Europe had demonstrated the bacterial basis of various infectious diseases. In the 1890s, the principle of immunization (beyond that from smallpox) was formulated, first for diphtheria. This greatly strengthened the capabilities of public health agencies in the control of communicable diseases.

The scope of health department functions did not broaden until the turn of the century, and the initiative was taken first by voluntary groups of citizens. Thus, in 1893, private philanthropy set up milk stations in New York City for poor mothers (who could not nurse their babies). The work of these stations gradually increased to include counseling of mothers on the general care of infants. Then, in 1908, the New York City Health Department organized a Bureau of Child Hygiene staffed by full-time nurses. These nurses visited the mothers of newborn babies in tenements, supervised midwives, inspected school children for detection of infectious disease, and conducted child health clinics. A National Association for Study and Prevention of Infant Mortality was formed in 1909 to promote such preventive child health programs throughout the United States.

Parallel developments led to the extension of health department activities to include the detection and follow-up of cases of tuberculosis. In 1892, the Pennsylvania Society for the Study and Prevention of Tuberculosis was founded, and by 1904 there were 23 such state and local associations. Among other things, special tuberculosis clinics were organized. In 1905, the Society for Social and Moral Prophylaxis was founded to encourage the prevention of venereal disease (VD), and VD clinics were set up. After the feasibility of these special clinics was demonstrated, public health agencies started similar programs. This greater scope of work strengthened the general image of health departments in the community.

In small towns when health departments were established, it was customary to designate some local physician as health officer. This physician would have the legal authority to enforce the regulations on sanitation and communicable diseases, although the day-to-day inspections and services were carried out by full-time sanitarians and nurses. In 1908, Jefferson County, Kentucky, appointed the first such full-time public health personnel to work throughout a county and outside city limits.

Thus, by 1910, public health agencies had become well established in state and local governments, although they had not yet acquired a major role in the overall health sector. The influence of voluntary agencies led to incremental expansion of public health functions beyond sanitary hygiene, but still within the sphere of prevention. Even the voluntary agencies were careful to emphasize their preventive objectives in order to avoid controversy with private physicians, who were expected to provide all medical treatment.

FOCUS ON PREVENTION, 1910–1935

The focus of public health agencies on preventive work was taken for granted; it was not a point of contention. Thus, when actions were taken to broaden the role of government on nonpreventive aspects of health, there was little reason to assign responsibilities to health departments. In

1910, the first law on worker's compensation for industrial accidents was enacted in New York State, soon to be followed by similar legislation in other states. Medical care was among the benefits of injured workers, but health departments were not involved; special new state agencies were established. Even when factory inspection programs were launched to assure safe working conditions, their implementation was assigned to a state department of labor or the like. Medical care of the poor was also sometimes a responsibility of local governments, but administration was done by departments of welfare concerned with other aspects of public assistance.

After 1910, various types of health service became increasingly organized, but the preventive focus of Health Departments ruled out any involvement by them. General hospitals were growing rapidly in number and overall bed capacity, so that a rising proportion of personal health care was given within their walls. Most hospitals were voluntary, but even public hospitals were seldom connected with health departments. Physicians were also increasing rapidly in number in the United States and were suspicious of competition from public agencies. Through their societies, they were always concerned about any governmental encroachment on their domain. Since local and even some state health officers were typically part-time private practitioners, they tended to share this attitude. This was reflected in various ways.

In the American Public Health Association (APHA) (founded in 1872), for example, a sociological section was organized in 1910. It was composed mainly of social workers concerned with the "social and economic aspects of health problems." Medical social work was taking shape in those years in order to help low-income patients coming to hospital outpatient departments and dispensaries. At this time the dominant group in the APHA were local health officers. (When a Committee on Municipal Public Health Practice was formed in 1920, it focused its attention solely on sanitation and quarantine—not even including maternal and child health services.) The American Medical Association (AMA), to which part-time local health officers typically belonged, was attacking all proposals to extend the health role of government. In this atmosphere, it is not surprising that by 1922 the APHA sociological section died a quiet death.

Conservatism in public health was particularly strong at the local government level. At the state level, there was greater likelihood for health departments to be directed by full-time professionals dedicated to a public health movement. Thus in 1916 the Conference of State and Territorial Health Officers discussed a number of proposals then in state legislatures to establish social insurance programs covering workers for medical care costs. (Great Britain had enacted general health insurance for workers in 1911, and the idea was discussed soon after in the United States—as an extension of the worker's compensation acts.) The state health officers gave support to these health insurance proposals and urged "close cooperation of the health insurance system with state, municipal and local health departments and boards." Local health officers, on the other hand, were reluctant to become concerned even with preventively oriented child health clinics.

In 1921, as a result of pressure from the labor movement and children's advocates, the Sheppard-Towner Act was passed by Congress; it established the first federal grants-in-aid for local child health clinics. The program was administered by the Children's Bureau, which had been established in 1912 in the federal Department of Labor (because of concern with banning child labor). Many local health departments, however, declined to accept these grants for fear of alienating private practitioners. The AMA and local medical societies opposed the program vigorously, and in 1928 Congress allowed it to terminate.

In some places, health officers were especially courageous and attempted to broaden the scope of public health work to include general medical services for the poor. In 1919, the Dawson committee in the British Ministry of Health advocated a network of health centers for both preventive and therapeutic ambulatory services. In 1920, a similar proposal was made by Herman Biggs, the health officer of New York State. The private medical profession, however, effectively killed this idea, as it killed a similar proposal by Dr. John Pomeroy, health officer of Los Angeles, a few years later.

By 1932, when the United States was into a deep economic depression and Franklin D. Roosevelt was elected president, the purely preventive focus of public health agencies was no longer challenged. In 1934, the Federal Emergency Relief Administration (FERA) gave the first federal grants to local government for public assistance to the poor, including financial support for medical care. The FERA funds were administered by welfare departments, and local health departments played no part. During this period the construction of public works was federally subsidized to provide jobs, and among other things many health centers were constructed. These facilities were used for housing health departments and their preventive clinics but never for the provision of medical care to the poor or other segments of the population.

The depression also caused a decline in the earnings of private physicians. As a result, many of them were glad to accept appointments as local health officers, often regarding this as a form of retirement. Dependence of local public health agencies almost entirely on meagre local government revenues inevitably meant very weak programs, even in the sphere of prevention. The quarters of most departments were typically in antiquated public buildings, with no links to hospitals or other medical facilities. Work in such settings naturally held little attraction for young physicians whose professional lives were ahead of them.

Thus, in the quarter-century between 1910 and 1935, public health agencies became widely established, but their scope was limited to environmental sanitation and preventive control of communicable diseases; the latter function had sometimes become extended to chronic disorders such as tuberculosis and venereal infection (their diagnosis but not treatment). In the overall arena of government, moreover, Health Departments were weak agencies, in comparison, for example, with boards of education or police departments.

The weakness of health departments was manifestly due to both internal and external causes. With untrained private physicians often in charge, there was little initiative to expand public health functions beyond traditional prevention. Even within government, health departments held little attraction as units for handling new or enlarged public tasks such as medical care of the poor; they commanded little respect. Yet without experience, how could they develop new capabilities? It was a vicious cycle.

EXPANSION AND DEVELOPMENT, 1935–1960

Enactment of the Social Security Act (SSA) in 1935 ushered in a very different period in U.S. public health. Early planning of this important legislation had considered the inclusion of a social insurance program for medical care—along with old-age pensions, unemployment compensation, and other benefits. But President Roosevelt did not want to jeopardize enactment of the entire law due to opposition from the medical profession. In place of health insurance, therefore, the act included two titles designed to strengthen public health services by federal grants-in-aid to the states.

Title V on the support of maternal and child health services (MCH) was essentially a resurrection and expansion of the old Sheppard-Towner act of 1921–1928. This title also authorized grants for the diagnosis and treatment of crippled children—clearly a nonpreventive task. Federal MCH activities came under the Children's Bureau in the Department of Labor, so that this program was handled separately from those for the rest of public health work. Title VI for general public health purposes came under the administration of the U.S. Public Health Service (USPHS), which had evolved in 1912 from the Marine Hospital Service. Because its historical origins had included tax collection from shipowners, the USPHS was, strangely enough, a part of the Treasury Department. In 1939, the USPHS, along with the Food and Drug Administration (FDA) (in the Department of Agriculture), the Social Security Board, and other related programs were brought together under the Federal Security Agency. These activities were not endowed with cabinet status until 1953, when the Department of Health, Education and Welfare (DHEW) was formed.

Federal grants to the states greatly strengthened public health agencies. State health departments everywhere acquired additional trained personnel, and local health departments were expanded. In fact, funds were earmarked to support formal training at university schools of public health. (These schools were also strengthened by the grants, and new schools were established.) Under Surgeon-General Thomas Parran, great emphasis was given to VD control, and hundreds of VD clinics were organized by local public health agencies. Since prevention of the spread of syphilis and gonorrhea required aggressive treatment of cases, this meant that health departments became engaged in personal medical care—if only for this disease category.

As health departments grew stronger, the perception of their proper responsibilities changed. State health departments, for example, developed services in industrial hygiene to study working conditions in industry in order to prevent occupational diseases. Local health departments undertook examinations of school children, often through agreements with boards of education. When World War II started in 1939, special attention was given to building up public health services in the vicinity of military training camps or in rapidly expanding war production areas. In order to promote community support for all sorts of public health activities, the field of health education took shape as a new professional discipline. Dental clinics were organized in health departments to do reparative work on the teeth of children and mothers seen in the MCH program (and in schools).

With the robust expansion of the entire field, there was much discussion about the proper scope of public health activities. The APHA was growing in membership and functions; one outcome was an important study directed by Haven Emerson (Dean of the Columbia University School of Public Health) and published in 1941, entitled "Local Health Units for the Nation." Among other things, this report emphasized that health departments should be concerned only with disease prevention. They should provide six basic services: environmental sanitation, communicable disease control, maternal and child health promotion (not treatment), laboratory services (in connection with disease prevention), vital statistics, and health education. This advocacy of the basic six tended to draw the lines in the public health movement between those who favored keeping the field confined to prevention and those who wanted to see it expanded to all aspects of the health of populations, including the planning and organization of medical care.

In the previous period, an important national study had been conducted by a prestigious Committee on the Costs of Medical Care (CCMC). The CCMC staff worked from 1928 to 1932, producing 27 volumes on all aspects of U.S. medical care, private and public. As a follow-up study in 1935–1936, the USPHS with the aid of the Works Progress Administration (WPA) conducted a National Health Survey that revealed a vast burden of untreated disease in the population, particularly in the lower income groups. Stimulated by these findings, Senator Robert Wagner (sponsor of the Social Security Act) introduced an amendment to this act in Congress, which would have supported federal grants to the states for the organization of health insurance plans covering workers and their dependents. This was in July 1939; the onset of World War II in September postponed any serious consideration of such an idea.

After the heavy involvement of the United States in Europe and the Pacific during World War II, work began on postwar planning. In 1943, new legislation was introduced in Congress for launching a federally administered national health insurance (NHI) program. This bill went through several versions, one of which assigned administrative responsibility to the USPHS. In support of the concept of public health agency participation in NHI administration, in 1944 the APHA governing council issued a now classic policy statement on Medical Care in a National Health Program. This action marked a turning point in the entire U.S. public health movement. The ideology of the old guard favoring only prevention was defeated and, at least among the most active leaders in the field, was replaced by the view that public health agencies should become concerned with all aspects of health service administration, including the delivery of medical care. In 1948, the APHA established a Medical Care Section, which soon became the largest group in the association.

In 1943, state health departments throughout the United States had been assigned a major new responsibility involving medical care administration. The Emergency Maternity and Infant Care (EMIC) program provided for governmental financing of maternity care (including childbirth) for the dependents of military personnel along with pediatric care of the infant during its first year of life. The EMIC program required the establishment of minimum standards for medical and hospital care, payment for these services, and related matters. Suddenly the state public health agencies found themselves heavily involved with responsibilities clearly beyond the boundaries of prevention.

After the war, another new and significant responsibility was delegated to state health departments. Although no NHI legislation was enacted, in 1946 the National Hospital Survey and Construction Act (Hill-Burton) became law. This federal program to subsidize the construction of hospitals in areas of bed shortage (mainly rural counties) had, in fact, been one section of a comprehensive NHI bill, which was separated and passed. Responsibility for surveying the hospital bed supply in each state and developing a master plan for new hospital construction where needed gave state public health agencies a wholly new type of experience. These agencies were also usually assigned the task of inspecting and licensing all hospitals and related facilities. (The nongovernmental Joint Commission on Accreditation of Hospitals was not established until 1952.)

In the postwar years, the scope and authority of public health agencies were also broadened in other ways. The National Mental Health Act (NMHA) became law in 1946 and provided grants to the states for research, prevention, diagnosis, and treatment of mental disorders. It was administered by a new branch of the USPHS and in most states mental health programs were developed in state health departments. At the local level, various types of mental health clinics were organized within health departments or other public and voluntary agencies.

These years also saw the entry of state and local health departments into the difficult field of chronic (noncommunicable) disease control. Heart disease and cancer had long been the major causes of death in the United States, and demands arose for some public health action. Accordingly, the early detection of chronic diseases became an objective of many public health agencies; mass population surveys with laboratory tests (e.g., blood glucose levels for identification of subclinical diabetes) were conducted. Eventually several such tests were performed on people at one time—a technique that became known as multiphasic screening. Public health agencies also began to promote rehabilitation services in hospitals and nursing homes. Some years later health education on lifestyle (diet, exercise, smoking, etc.) became a customary public health activity for the purpose of preventing heart disease and cancer.

During the 1950s there was further expansion of public health activities at the federal level. The National Institutes of Health (NIH) within the USPHS were greatly expanded for the support of biomedical research both intramurally and through grants to universities and other places. In 1954, the operation of a comprehensive health service for American Indians was transferred from the Department of Interior to the USPHS. In 1956 Congress authorized the USPHS to conduct a continuing national health survey for the identification of every kind of illness in the population and the types and amounts of medical care received by families.

By the end of this period (1960), the scope and importance of federal, state, and local public health agencies had clearly become far greater than in 1935. Although organized health activities had also expanded under other types of sponsorship—welfare departments, public and private hospitals, voluntary health insurance organizations—health departments were participating actively in the extension of social responsibilities for health. Furthermore, under innovative leadership, some health departments assumed unusually broad responsibilities, such as administration of the medical care program for the poor (public assistance recipients) in Maryland or the combined responsibility for public health and public hospitals in Denver, Colorado.

HEALTH CARE PROGRESS
ELSEWHERE, 1960–1980

In the 1960s, governmental responsibilities for various aspects of health continued to expand, although principally in organizations other than departments of health. The 1963 Health Professions Educational Assistance Act was administered federally by the USPHS, but the grants went entirely to universities and colleges, without any involvement of state or local health departments. In response to a sort of rediscovery of poverty, the federal Economic Opportunity Act (EOA) was passed in 1964. President Johnson spoke of declaring a war on poverty, and the EOA established a new U.S. Office of Economic Opportunity (OEO) outside the DHEW and reporting directly to the president. In 1965, the OEO launched a program of federal support for neighborhood health centers in impoverished sections of cities and rural areas. These facilities offered poor people a comprehensive range of ambulatory medical services, both therapeutic and preventive.

A special feature of OEO health centers was maximum community participation, meaning the participation of poor people themselves in the determination of policies and administrative practices. Between 1965 and 1971 about 100 neighborhood health centers were established. Although local health departments played a role in the origins of a few of these centers, by 1971 not a single center had any connection with a public health agency.

In 1973, under President Nixon, the OEO was terminated and its neighborhood health centers were transferred to the supervision of the USPHS. In the meantime, several other types of community health centers (as these facilities came to be called) were launched under various new federal grant programs—aggregating to nearly 1000 such facilities by 1979. In spite of their USPHS federal supervision, very few of these units involved any health department management. The vast majority were operated by newly formed local nongovernmental community organizations. Many facilities were related in some way to hospitals or medical schools, but not to departments of health.

This explosive development of community health centers for the poor did, however, have an influence on local health departments, especially those in large cities. The popularity of comprehensive health services offered in free-standing facilities convinced some public health agencies to broaden the scope of their traditional categorical clinics. Instead of limiting their functions to preventive MCH services or to treating VD, health department clinics began to offer general primary medical care.

A turning point came in 1965, when SSA amendments launched the major health programs soon labeled as Medicare and Medicaid. The problem of financing medical care for the aged had been evident for some years; a greater burden of sickness had to be faced in the later years of life just when most people lost their voluntary insurance coverage because of retirement from work (such insurance being linked so often to employment). The Medicare program gave health insurance protection to people eligible for old-age pensions under SSA. Although some personal cost-sharing was required, most medical and hospitalization costs were met by the government.

The other population group with little protection by voluntary health insurance was the poor. The Medicaid program, depending on both federal and state general revenues, financed a broad range of services for public assistance recipients and certain other medically indigent people. Both Medicare and Medicaid were essentially payment mechanisms for services in the medical mainstream, that is, services from private physicians, community hospitals, and other health care providers serving the population as a whole.

Medicare and Medicaid rapidly became the largest programs for health purposes in the federal government. Their costs soon dwarfed expenditures for all other governmental health-related programs combined. In the administration of these major programs, however, public health agencies at federal, state, and local levels played almost no part. Under Medicare, payments were handled by fiscal intermediaries drawn from Blue Cross and Blue Shield plans and commercial insurance companies. Medicaid was most often managed by state welfare agencies or new bodies established in state governments. Occasionally the state health department was administratively involved, but the local health departments never were. About 1975, a new agency was set up under the federal DHEW solely for Medicare and Medicaid management—the Health Care Financing Administration.

In late 1965, another important federal health program was started; it was to promote improvement in the quality of medical care through various regionalized educational and consultative activities. To make the law politically attractive, it was linked to the three greatest causes of death in the United States (mainly in old people) and designated as the Regional Medical Program for Heart Disease, Cancer and Stroke (RMP). At the federal level RMP was administered by the USPHS, but no role was played by public health agencies at state or local levels. By 1972, federal RMP grants went to 56 organizations that blanketed the United States; of these, 33 were sponsored by universities, 4 by medical societies, and 19 by other new or existent corporate bodies. Not a single RMP program came under a state or local health department.

In 1966, the first U.S. law on Comprehensive Health Planning (CHP) was enacted. The CHP agencies were to be organized in every state and local area "to support the marshalling of all health resources—national, state, and local—to assure comprehensive health services of high quality for every person." At the state level the governor was to appoint a State Health Planning Council, and in about half the cases this was in the state health department. At the local level, 198 areawide CHP agencies had been established by 1972; of these, 150 were new private nonprofit organizations, 45 were special quasigovernmental district councils, and only 3 had any relationship to local health departments. The principal work of CHP agencies was hospital planning, but their scope theoretically encompasses all organized health activities. One can hardly think of a role more suitable for local public health agencies to perform, but this was almost never the case.

The last straw in the legislative bypassing of public health agencies was the enactment of the National Health Planning and Resources Development Act of 1974. This legislation replaced both the RMP and CHP laws with a nationwide planning program of very broad scope. Once again federal administration was assigned to the USPHS, but at the state level only about half the governors designated the state health department as the administrative agency. More important, by 1979 at the local level, 203 Health Systems Agencies (HSA) were established, of which 178 were private nonprofit entities. Only 25 HSAs were established in any branch of local government, not necessarily involving the local health department. The language of the federal law, in fact, made it difficult for local health departments to play this crucial planning role.

Other types of health care organization developed in the United States during 1960–1980. The Health Maintenance Organization (HMO) Act of 1973 provided for federal promotion of these special forms of medical service, which organized both the financing and delivery of comprehensive health services in a manner that yielded economies. In 1975, further amendments of the SSA established a nationwide network of Professional Standards Review Organizations (PSRO) to monitor the services provided under Medicare and Medicaid.

Both HMOs and PSROs functioned essentially at the community level, but the local health department was almost never involved. Still other important movements for the increased organization of services, such as voluntary health insurance and private group medical practice, were entirely outside the domain of government.

Another health feature of the 1970s was a reopened legislative debate on a national health insurance program. In part because of Medicare and Medicaid, which pumped more money into the health sector without changing patterns of health care delivery, medical care costs rose very rapidly, becoming increasingly burdensome to the average family. Numerous proposals were introduced in Congress, therefore, to extend economic support of medical costs from the aged and the poor to the total population. The various bills differed in their scope and degree of impact on patterns of health care, but (as in the 1940s) legislative agreement could not be reached on any of them. In the late 1970s, in part due to the stalemate on health insurance and in part due to research findings on the role of personal lifestyle in the development of chronic disease, the federal government shifted its priorities. There was a kind of rediscovery of the importance of prevention and health promotion. Thus the health education component of public health programs got a major boost, but this was in the traditional sphere of prevention.

Thus in the period 1960–1980, the long-term trend toward greater organization of health services continued and even accelerated. In terms of dollars spent in an organized framework, including voluntary health insurance and government at all levels, by 1977 nearly 70 percent of health services involved third parties. In terms of the services delivered to people, a rising proportion was being provided in hospitals—inherently very organized settings compared with physicians' offices. Even ambulatory health care was becoming increasingly organized through diverse types of clinics under both governmental and private sponsorship. Very few of these developments, however, involved public health agencies.

GENERAL INTERPRETATION

We have now considered five periods in the evolution of public health activities in the United States. In the first period (1800–1870), community responsibility began to be taken for the health of populations, mainly in cities in which concentrations of people created greater health hazards. Boards of health were appointed to formulate rules and regulations on environmental sanitation to reduce those hazards. In the second period (1870–1910), public health agencies with full-time civil servants became established as a normal part of state and local governments; then, largely through the influence of voluntary organizations, the scope of these governmental agencies gradually broadened beyond sanitation and the control of the acute communicable diseases.

In the third period (1910–1935), many other forms of organization of the health sector took place. At the same time, private medical practitioners became more important in the average community: they implemented the advancing medical science and commanded great respect. As small businesses selling services for patient fees, however, physicians were much concerned about the encroachment of governmental health programs on their domain. To avoid controversy and opposition from the medical profession, therefore, state and local health departments were careful to confine their activities to disease prevention. Medical diagnosis and treatment were regarded as the exclusive prerogative of private physicians.

The fourth period (1935–1960) was marked by a deep economic depression, a destructive world war, and expansion of the role of government in many spheres. In these circumstances, public health agencies at all levels—federal, state, and local—increased greatly in strength and scope. Although their principal role remained the prevention of disease, health departments (especially at state and federal levels) acquired new responsibilities in medical care administration. The definition of the term "prevention" was also broadened to include the early detection of patients with chronic disease, rehabilitation of the physically handicapped, and ambulatory care of patients with mental disorders.

The fifth period (1960–1980) brought further expansion of organized programs in the health sector. Most of the action took place, however, outside the sphere of government or, if in government, under agencies other than health departments. Large new social programs—Medicare, Medicaid, RMP, CHP, HMO promotion, and so on—greatly enlarged the share of total health expenditures coming under some type of organized arrangements. Public health agencies did not actually decline in their resources and services, but the major social developments in the health sector occurred in other places. Compared to the blossoming of health departments in the previous period, there seemed to be a *relative* decline in their stature in 1960–1980.

What can be identified to account for these changing trends? It is evident that U.S. health care has become increasingly subject to regulation, planning, and social controls over at least the last century. This has been generally opposed by the private sector of U.S. health services, including not only most physicians and dentists but voluntary hospitals, pharmaceutical companies, and even professional schools as well. All these groups tended to view with alarm the expanding power of government and the diminishing independence of the private health sector.

If these trends could not be stopped, at least their impact could be weakened. Conservatism in the health care system was inevitably mirrored in the halls of the U.S. Congress. The strategy may not have been so crude and deliberate as the military policy of divide and conquer, but its effects were the same. No single public agency would be permitted to become very powerful. Insofar as authority was to be delegated below the national level, it should be dispersed. Medical schools, as well as hospitals, insurance carriers, welfare departments, or wholly new nongovernmental bodies, should play a part. The long history and the established legal status of public health agencies should not be permitted to endow them with a central role in the health sector. Broad authorities in any single type of state or local agency would constitute a continuing threat to the independence of the private sector.

There have also been weaknesses in the caliber of public health personnel. The decade of 1935–1945 was a time of great social change in the United States; it attracted into government many idealists and fighters for improvement in society. By the 1950s, with conservative national governments and the cold war atmosphere in the world, things were different. Physicians and others entering public health tried, in the main, to avoid controversy and to keep the agency on an even keel, not to tackle unmet social needs. The crusaders of the New Deal period were replaced by a cohort of office holders and managers.

The 1960s and 1970s in the United States then brought a new generation of young activists eager for social change, but few of them entered public health work. Health departments, like other parts of government, were seen as representing the status quo; the most spirited young people wanted to work in the community without bureaucratic restraint. Public health agencies did not enjoy the swelling flow of financial support they had in the previous period; the principal innovations were occurring in other parts of the health care system. Assignment of health planning responsibilities to wholly new agencies (mainly nongovernmental, in spite of their federal public support) was a particular blow to the public health movement.

Thus, circumstances in the national environment, as well as in the internal staffing of health departments, contributed to the modest role these agencies played in the U.S. health sector of the 1960s and 1970s. Relatively few voices from the public health movement were heard in reaction to the great fragmentation of organized health programs. Aggressive leadership demanding social reforms in the U.S. health sector was replaced by the posture of the low profile.

With the election of the conservative Republican administration in 1981, there has been increasing pressure for termination, if not reversal, of past trends—less social planning and regulation, a smaller public sector and a larger private sector in health as in other aspects of life, and an abrupt reduction in governmental financing for social programs, particularly at the federal level. In the case of public regulations, a major effort has been made to reduce their impact on the health services, if not eliminate them entirely. The central thrust has been to maximize private health services and minimize regulatory controls, transferring responsibilities whenever possible from the federal to the state and local levels.

At this point, one can, of course, only speculate about the future. Will the whole structure of organized health services in the United States continue to go downhill? Or will a reaction set in to reestablish public responsibility for health services in general and public health activities in particular? If a reconstruction period should occur in the later 1980s, one might even expect that health departments—with their long tradition in local, state, and federal governments—may regain a central position in the structure of government, with major responsibilities for the planning and delivery of health services in the United States.

GENERAL REFERENCES

Jain SC (ed): "Role of state and local governments in relation to personal health services." American Journal of Public Health, January 1981: 71, Supplement.

Jonas S, et al: Health Care Delivery in the United States. New York: Springer Publishing Co, 1977.

Last JM (ed): Maxcy-Rosenau: Public Health and Preventive Medicine (11th ed.) New York: Appleton-Century-Crofts, 1980.

Mustard HS: Government in Public Health. New York: Commonwealth Fund, 1945.

Rosen G: A History of Public Health. New York: MD Publications, 1958.

Silver GA: A Spy in the House of Medicine. Germantown, Md.: Aspen Systems Corp., 1976.

Chapter 4

Nursing and Developments in Other Health Professions*

Health manpower was discussed briefly in Chapter 1, but here we examine more thoroughly this crucial aspect of every national health system. Special attention must be given to nursing, which has been undergoing particularly great changes in the United States, and is the largest of the health professions.

THE DIVERSITY OF HEALTH MANPOWER

In 1982 there were 7,863,000 people employed in the health care system of the United States, comprising about 7 percent of the active work force of the nation. Classified by the places where they work, much the largest proportion of health personnel are in hospitals.[1] Their distribution in 1982 was as follows:

Place of Work	Percent
Hospitals	55.2
Convalescent facilities	15.5
Physician's offices or clinics	11.4
Dental offices	5.3
Offices of other health practitioners	1.7
Other health services sites	10.9
All places	100.0

*The major section entitled "The Largest Health Profession: Nursing," was written by Donna F. Ver Steeg, R.N., Ph.D., F.A.A.N., Assoc. Prof. of Nursing, Univ. of California, Los Angeles.

By far the largest category of health personnel are nurses of all levels. These numbered about 2,500,000 in 1980 or about one-third of the total health manpower; the several levels of nurse and developments in nursing are discussed later.

The complexity of the U.S. health care system is reflected by the ratio of various health personnel to physicians. In 1982, when there were about 480,000 active physicians, there were about 16 other health personnel for each doctor. This compares with about 3 other health personnel per doctor in 1920.[2] The great majority of these "other personnel" have skills acquired through special training, and only about one-fifth might be considered nonspecific clerical or custodial or similar personnel.

Among the skilled health personnel, the categories are so numerous that the U.S. Department of Labor has identified as many as 700 different types. Aside from nurses and physicians, the most numerous are pharmacists, dentists, and laboratory technicians or technologists. Beyond these are several types of practitioner who, under the laws of most U.S. states, may serve patients directly—that is, without supervision by a doctor. These include chiropractors, optometrists, podiatrists, and, in a few states, midwives. Each of these health personnel types number in the thousands. Osteopaths were once considered a "healing cult," similar to chiropractors (who attempt to treat all disorders by manipulating the vertebral column), but they have now evolved along scientific lines, which warrants their inclusion in the count of physicians.

The types and numbers of health personnel who work along with physicians, under their direct or indirect supervision, are much greater. Conceptually, these "allied" health personnel work on teams with physicians, although in practice the teamwork may be quite amorphous. Beyond the types of health professionals mentioned above, there are numerous technicians outside the clinical laboratory, such as x-ray technicians, electrocardiograph technicians, technicians trained in operating special equipment such as kidney dialysis machines, and so on. In rehabilitation service there are physical, occupational, and speech therapists. In mental health services, aside from psychiatrists, there are psychologists, psychiatric social workers, and psychiatric nurses. For dental care, aside from dentists, there are dental hygienists, dental technicians, and dental assistants. Other special tasks are performed by nutritionists and dietitians, by statisticians and statistical clerks, by medical record librarians and information system specialists. For very specialized roles, there are respiratory therapists, audiologists, and plaster cast technicians.

In contrast to this specialization of functions, the nurse is a broad generalist. Many of the functions of the personnel noted above were done, in previous times, by physicians and nurses. In countries less developed than the United States, the work of the laboratory technician, physical therapist, or dietitian may at present be done by the nurse. The structure and functions of nursing in the United States warrant more thorough examination.

THE LARGEST HEALTH PROFESSION: NURSING

Nursing now constitutes the largest single group in the health professional work force of the United States. It has achieved this numerical dominance primarily as a result of the rapid increase in hospital medical technology. Because of the rapidly increasing cost of this technology, future changes in the number and preparation of nurses are expected to reflect a shift from hospital care to convalescent care, home care, and nursing homes. There is no expectation that the numbers of nurses will decrease in comparison with other health professionals.

Numbers and Categories of Nurses

The 1910 U.S. Census reported little more than half as many trained nurses as physicians and surgeons.[3] Even with the addition of nurses (untrained) and midwives, the total nursing personnel in 1910 numbered less than 1.5 times the number of physicians and surgeons.[3, 4] By 1980, there were almost 2.5 times as many registered nurses as physicians. Counting all levels of nursing (registered nurses, licensed practical nurses, nurses aides, orderlies, and attendants) there were 6.8 times as many nursing personnel as physicians. Considering only registered nurses, they increased from 55 per 100,000 population in 1910 to 502 per 100,000 in 1980.[5]

Within these national ratios, however, is a considerable variation across geographic areas and between rural and urban and underserved areas. In 1977, the registered nurse ratios varied from 332 per 100,000 in the South to 503 per 100,000 in the Northeast. Ratios for licensed practical nurses varied in 1974 from 149 per 100,000 in the West to 186 per 100,000 in the South.[6]

The educational preparation for nursing practice has been multi-tiered. One cannot assume from the term "nurse" alone a given level of competence. Registered nurses (RNs) are licensed by the state to practice professional nursing. They must be high school graduates and receive their prelicensure education in a hospital-based diploma program, a college or university-based baccalaureate program (BSN), or, since 1952, in a junior college-based associate degree program (ADN). Registered nurses may receive formal advanced education either in college- or university-based master's and doctoral programs. Increasingly, these advanced practitioners are also certified by governmental and/or professional bodies.

Policy planning for nurse manpower has been hampered by the fact that two of the largest data systems, the U.S. Census and the American Hospital Association annual hospital survey, do not distinguish between levels of registered nurse education. Other surveys, such as those by the American Nurses Association and the National League for Nursing, have collected different data in different years.[7, 8]

Licensed practical nurses (LPNs), called licensed vocational nurses (LVNs) in two states, are nurses who may or may not have completed high school before entering a one-year program. LPN/LVN programs may be operated by a variety of organizations including adult schools, junior colleges, and technical schools. Like RNs, LPN/LVNs must pass a state-supervised examination to become licensed. Licensed practical nurses work under the general supervision of registered nurses.

Nurse's aides, orderlies, home health aides, and attendants usually work under the supervision of licensed nurses. They may or may not undergo a short formal educational program in addition to on-the-job training. The "mix" of RNs, LPN/LVNs, aides, orderlies, and so on depends on the nature of the patient care provided by the employing organization. Sometimes the mix is determined by governmental regulation and sometimes by the budget. Financial incentives have been provided in some state legislation to encourage facilities, such as nursing homes, to employ better qualified nursing staff.

Work Settings

Nurses work in a variety of settings, but over the years the principal trend has been from private practice (or private service to patients in hospitals or at home) to hospital employment. However, the new Diagnosis Related Groups (DRG) hospital reimbursement program, applied recently in most states to contain Medicare costs, has resulted in a lessening of this trend. Statistics are not yet available on how this has affected employment patterns, but hospitals are now under fiscal pressure to move patients out of the hospital sooner, resulting in greater emphasis on out-of-hospital care. Before 1915, the great majority of hospital nurses were students and the great majority of graduate nurses were self-employed in private duty. In 1928, less than one-fourth of all trained nurses were employed in hospitals. After World War II, the trend toward hospital employment and the decline in private practice continued. The distribution of work settings and the trends from 1949 to 1980 are shown in Table 4.1.

More than 80 percent of licensed practical nurses also work in hospitals and nursing homes. The relative proportion of RNs and LPN/LVNs working in hospitals varies both geographically and between types and sizes of hospitals. Lower percentages of LPN/LVNs are found in short-term general hospitals and hospitals of more than 500 beds. The highest percentage of LPN/LVNs are found in long-term hospitals and hospitals of 25–49 beds. Higher percentages of LPN/LVNs are also found in the South Atlantic and East North Central states, with the lowest percentages in New England and the Mountain States.[8]

Table 4.1. Work Settings of Active Registered Nurses: Percentage Distribution in Selected Years

Work Setting	1949	1962	1980
Hospitals and nursing homes	47.2	63.0	73.6
Public health/schools	9.5	7.6	10.1
Occupational health	4.4	3.3	2.3
Nursing education	4.0	3.1	3.7
Office nurses	8.8	12.1	5.7
Private duty, self-employed, and other	22.2	8.7	4.2
Unclassified	3.9	2.2	0.6
All settings	100.0	100.0	100.0

Traditionally there were no salary differences for hospital staff nurses, based on education and experience. This is changing, however, largely because state nurses associations began to function as unions to represent their members and bargain collectively with employers. Discrepancies between the salaries of male and female nurses, as in other health professions, remain a problem, as shown in Table 4.2.[5]

With the advent of widespread collective bargaining for nurses in 1974, it became possible for more nurses to plan for retirement in the same way as other workers. As a result, the ranks of inactive nurses include a larger proportion of older nurses than formerly. At the same time younger nurses, who once left the work force during their childbearing years, are more likely to remain employed on at least a part-time basis. Over 70 percent of working RNs are married and only 14 percent have never been married. Nevertheless, the active employment rate for nursing is much higher than for the population (male and female) as a whole.

Definition of Nursing

In 1960, the International Congress of Nurses adopted a statement on the basic definition of nursing. This statement has served as the basis for some of the most forward-looking state nurse practice acts in the United States. According to the ICN statement:

> The unique function of the nurse is to assist the individual sick or well in the performance of those activities contributing to health or its recovery (or a peaceful death) that he would perform unaided if he had the necessary strength, will or knowledge. And to do this in such a way as to help him gain independence as rapidly as possible. . . .

Table 4.2. Mean Annual Earnings of Health Personnel, by Sex, 1979

Personnel	Male	Female
Physicians	$60,247	$31,637
Registered nurses	19,122	14,834
Physician's assistants	16,054	10,542
Licensed practical nurses	12,807	10,341
Nurse's aides, orderlies, and attendants	12,124	8,433

The California Nurse Practice Act, extensively rewritten in 1974 and subsequently amended, defines nursing as:

> Those functions, including basic health care, which help people cope with difficulties in daily living, which are associated with their actual or potential health or illness problems or the treatment thereof, [and] which require a substantial amount of scientific knowledge or technical skill. . . .

Nurse educators and researchers, now better prepared for their scholarly tasks, maintain that the essential nature of nursing has not changed. It is the ability to describe and define nursing practice that is changing. Nationally, nurses in practice and academia refer to nursing diagnoses in measurable and reproducible terms. Such diagnoses are defined in terms of human behavior, for which there are nursing interventions as distinct from medical interventions. Thus nurses are concerned with such problems as patients' inability to care for themselves without help, nutritional deficits or excesses, and inadequate coping strategies. Each diagnosis is described in terms of etiology, defining characteristics, and expectations for nursing interventions.[9]

Changing from intuitive to scientifically defensible practice allows for a new level of nurse autonomy and accountability. Identifiable and measurable services pave the way for different types of payment for nursing, and create the opportunity for new working environments for nursing practice. Problems covered by nursing diagnoses are frequently those which also extend hospital stay. The interaction of nursing diagnoses and DRGs is likely to provide the basis for a more accurate formula for predicting hospital costs and reimbursements. This should lead to much greater recognition of the importance of good nursing care.

Registered nursing is one of the relatively few college-level occupations that is expected to continue to grow in numbers in the next 20 years. The roles and functions of nurses will change as hospitals stress intensive care and more patients are shifted to home care. The increasing age of the population will create greater demands for nursing services. More and more nurses will be working in environments where direct supervision by others is not feasible. This will require a broader mandate in ambulatory care, analogous to the changing role of hospital nursing with the development of 24-hour intensive care units in the 1960s.

Much has been said about the supposed competition between nurses and physicians, as the numbers of physicians increase. There is no evidence to support the idea that physicians can replace nurses, but it is very likely that much of the work currently done by physicians-in-training in hospitals and clinics will be taken over by nurses. How much impact this continuing change in responsibility will have on nurse authority remains to be seen. It is not likely that the professional nurses of the 1980s and beyond will be willing to take on one without the other.

Nursing Education

Nursing in the United States first became a discipline for formal training in 1873. By 1910, many hospitals depended on their own nursing schools for low-cost labor. Often there was little concern for the quality of the student's education. Lectures, when they were not canceled, were held after long hours of work. Libraries and laboratories, if they existed at all, were inadequate. Direct supervision of the younger student's clinical experience depended heavily on senior students. Some hospitals hired out students for private-duty nursing in patients' homes, to increase hospital earnings.[10]

Concern about the poor quality of these programs eventually led to a national study, the Goldmark Report, published in 1923. This report revealed that, while there were some good schools, the average hospital was not equipped to provide more than a casual education, poorly related to the students' clinical experience. The health of students was being damaged by the conditions under which they lived, worked, and studied. While the report recognized the key role of hospitals in the clinical training of nurses, it strongly recommended that the educational process be under the control of educational institutions. Colleges and universities were better equipped to provide the necessary libraries, laboratories, classrooms, and instructors in the basic sciences required for professional-level education.[10]

A similar report by Flexner on medical education a few years earlier had resulted in the fairly rapid closure of substandard schools of medicine and the infusion of private and public funds to upgrade medical education. It took several decades and a national emergency, however, before nursing was able to develop the resources needed for improving nursing education. One must keep in mind that women achieved the right to vote only in 1920, and the education of women was not a high priority during this period.

With the onset of World War II, Congress became concerned about the shortage of registered nurses. In 1942, legislation was passed authorizing the Cadet Nurse Corps. Nursing leaders could at last develop and enforce standards for the accreditation of school facilities, faculties, and curricula. The federal government provided funds to assist schools in meeting these standards. The magnitude of the task faced was shown in the Brown Report of 1948. Some 97 percent of nursing schools were found to be still under hospital control, and few nurses were prepared academically to hold faculty positions in colleges and universities.[10]

Prior to 1950, there were only nine doctorally prepared nurses in the United States. By 1980, a national survey identified 3650 nurses with doctorates.[8] A survey of nursing faculties as late as 1982, however, indicated that 22 percent of the teachers in Associate Degree programs and 49 percent of the teachers in hospital diploma programs lack even a master's degree. Among baccalaureate nursing programs, only 16 percent of the faculty held doctorates. Among the faculty of LPN/LVN programs, 51.2 percent were prepared at the baccalaureate level in nursing and 21.5 percent were diploma graduates.[7]

The long delay in supporting an academic base retarded the whole development of nursing. Nursing became one of the least educated professions. By 1979, three-fourths of all women in professional/technical employment had four or more years of college education. Only one-fourth of registered nurses had that much education. Nurses with associate degree or diploma education constituted three-fourths of the profession in 1980.[8, 5] It should be noted that 17.7 percent of all unemployed women with some college are registered nurses.[5]

Much of the opposition to academically based programs has come from within the nursing profession itself. Only in the early 1980s was the concensus reached across all of the major national nursing organizations that nursing education belonged in an academic setting. It was finally agreed that entry into practice at the professional level would require the baccalaureate degree and, at the technical level, the associate degree.

Formal preparation and licensure for practical nurses had become widespread in the early 1950s during a nursing shortage following

World War II. In 1984, LPN programs nationally became committed to extending their training to 18 months. They would then become the technical nurses envisioned as the second category of nurses by the major registered nursing organizations. The markedly changed structure of nursing education is shown in Table 4.3.[7]

The remaining diploma programs in hospitals are gradually affiliating with universities or colleges for curriculum control and for granting of academic degrees. Not shown in the table are the post-RN baccalaureate programs. These provide educational access for registered nurses already holding diplomas or associate degrees. In 1980, there were 117,000 RNs enrolled in baccalaureate degree programs.[7]

Nursing Functions

The practice of nursing has long had to overcome social objections to a person's intimate access to the bodies of strangers of both sexes. Traditionally, such access was permissible only for healers and for servants. Healing implied great learning, command of secret knowledge, and special tools. Many of the common visible clinical skills of nursing are viewed as parenting in nature and menial. These skills are viewed as requiring mainly common sense to perform. They are regarded as within the competence of untrained servants or dedicated volunteers.

The basic fallacy of the latter viewpoint has been repeatedly recognized. When Florence Nightingale traveled in 1854 to the Turkish Crimea, in response to a governmental mandate to improve hospital care, her first problem was selecting qualified nurses. Her second problem was to convince the military physicians that the care she and her nurses proposed to provide would not spoil the soldiers by "coddling the brutes." The nursing reforms eventually reduced in-hospital mortality

Table 4.3. Graduations from Prelicensure RN Schools of Nursing by Degree: Percentage Distribution, 1952 to 1982

Educational Credential	1952	1962	1972	1982
Associate degree	1.0	3.7	37.0	51.7
Diploma (hospital schools)	92.1	82.5	41.7	15.8
Baccalaureate degree	6.9	13.8	21.3	32.5

from 60 percent to little more than 1 percent, but this did not prevent repeated attempts to undermine the program and eliminate the nurses. In the United States, soldiers in the Spanish American War and World War I suffered, while nurses struggled for the right to provide qualified nursing care. It was not until 1944 that nurses in the military forces were granted temporary status as officers. Only in 1947 did Congress establish permanent Army and Navy Nurse Corps.[10]

Several types of nursing activity have developed over the years. In 1902, the value of school nursing in maintaining the health and attendance of school children was first demonstrated in New York City. Yet even in the 1980s, when school budgets have been reduced, school nurses have often been terminated before football coaches. The early experience in the schools of New York led the Metropolitan Life Insurance Company to set up a "visiting nursing service" for its industrial policyholders. This service, with the slogan "Call for a nurse when you need to be nursed," was highly successful in reducing health problems among insured families; it was continued until 1950, when other equivalent services became available.[10]

Nurse midwives, who care for normal mothers throughout the childbearing cycle, have demonstrated consistently in the United States and in other countries that their care reduces infant and maternal morbidity and mortality significantly. Despite this evidence, nurse midwives have had great difficulty in practicing in the United States because of restrictive licensing and reimbursement policies and the opposition of the medical profession.[11]

The crucial importance of qualified nursing care in the hospital environment has been repeatedly demonstrated. One of the causes of increased hospital costs has been the overuse of intensive care units for patients not needing such technology. These patients are sent by physicians who want the closer nursing supervision possible in such units.[11]

Nurses in Expanded Roles

Nurses have traditionally expanded their practice through on-the-job training and only later formalized such preparation in an educational program. Thus, the first public health nurses in World War I, the first maternal and child health nurses in the early 1920s, the first nurse anesthetists, nurse midwives, clinical nurse specialists, and nurse practitioners were all prepared outside the formal educational system. In each instance, however, these initial efforts were followed by the establishment of standards, formal curricula in approved programs, and more recently, the preparation for advanced levels through master's degree programs in universities. Usually, the initial programs were federally funded in an attempt to meet some major public health problem facing the country. Often these programs initially required waivers of state laws restricting nursing practice, because they exposed what had previously been covert nursing practice. The principles and content of nursing had not changed, but the public recognition of its scope had.

Over time, the acceptance of nursing's role as shown in actual practice has led to changes in nurse practice laws across the country. These changes have led to challenges in the courts from threatened members of other health professions. Since differences have not been demonstrated in the quality of care provided by qualified nurses and physicians, the ultimate battle will probably concern the issue of restraint of trade. There is good evidence that much of normal pregnancy and delivery, much of primary ambulatory care, and much of straightforward anesthesia can be provided at least as well by properly prepared nurses in advanced practice as by physicians. Physician control over access to care, through licensure and reimbursement for services, is therefore being challenged as an economic issue and against the public interest.[11]

In 1980, there were some 50,400 registered nurses employed in advanced practice positions as nurse practitioners, nurse midwives, clinical nurse specialists, and nurse anesthetists. Of these, 8.8 percent received their preparation in master's degree programs and 22 percent had no formal preparation, but had qualified through on-the-job training and examinations. Recently enacted legislation in many states provides for review of the qualifications of these practitioners by the state Boards of Nursing.[8]

With knowledge and experience, some clinical procedures originally reserved for advanced nursing practitioners are being incorporated into basic nursing education. The changed appearance of common nursing practice has led to changes in relationships and mutual expectations of nurses and other health professionals. The nurse's use of the special tools formerly reserved for physicians began with thermometers, proceeded to hypodermic syringes, blood pressure cuffs in World War II, and now includes such items as venipuncture needles, otoophthalmoscopes, blood gas analyzers, and cardiac defibrillation equipment for cardiac arrest. The use of each new tool by nurses has usually been seen as a threat by physicians, until the advantages have been demonstrated.

Men in Nursing

Intricately interwoven with the healer/servant dilemma for nursing has been the issue of women and "women's tasks." How convoluted this all becomes is illustrated by the fact that as late as 1980, a male registered nurse was forbidden to work in a labor and delivery room with new mothers, although most of the attending obstetricians were men.

Men were not well treated in nursing after the turn of the century. They were usually restricted to men-only programs and restricted as well in the clients they served. The percentage of men in nursing is still small. Prior to 1966, men were not eligible for appointment to the Army, Navy, and Air Force Nurse Corps. This restriction had its most dramatic effect on the number of men in nursing during World War II when they nearly disappeared. Male nurses were drafted to serve as corpsmen and pharmacists mates—not nurses. Male student nurses did not receive deferments to complete their nursing education.[10] It took a number of years for men in nursing to regain the losses suffered during this period. By 1981, however, 7.54 percent of the graduates of all basic RN programs in the United States were men. In some states (Alaska, Missouri, and Oregon) and in Puerto Rico, more than 10 percent of the graduates that year were men.[7]

Using 1980 Census figures, men constitute only about 4 percent of the overall supply of RNs, 3.4 percent of the LPN/LVNs, and 12.5 percent of nurse's aides, orderlies, and attendants.[5]

The participation of minority ethnic groups has historically been limited in the nursing profession, as in other professions. Social prejudice against certain ethnic groups and by members of certain minority groups against nursing was strong.

Inadequate prenursing education and other social conditions contributed to this problem. In 1980, when the population of the United States was 14.1 percent ethnic minorities, only 7.2 percent of RNs were from such groups. The enforcement of civil rights legislation and the initiative of professional organizations has improved this situation somewhat. As a group, minority RNs are actually better prepared academically than the RN population as a whole. Among LPN/LVNs there is a much higher percentage of minority group members. Among less skilled nursing personnel, the percentage is even higher.

Physician's Assistants

Physician's assistants (PAs) are a recently defined category of health manpower, developed originally for ex-medical corpsmen of the Vietnam War. They were created in the late 1960s as a response to the shortage of physicians in rural and underserved areas, and the unwillingness of nurses to assume responsibility without authority. Over time the supply of corpsmen has diminished, and current PA students are recruited from the ranks of a number of health-related occupations. Some PAs are also registered nurses, but they are not separately licensed. They are required to pass a national certifying examination, but they practice under the authority of their supervising physician. Nurse practitioners, who are often compared to PAs, are all registered nurses. In many states they also carry advanced certification which allows them to prescribe medication and charge fees for their services.

NEW TRENDS IN MEDICINE

The great extent of specialization in the American medical profession has been noted earlier. In 1981, out of 426,000 professionally active physicians, only about 49,000 or 11.5 percent were in office-based general practice or in the newly defined specialty of "family practice." The rise of the latter specialty was a significant reaction to the excessive specialization that had taken shape in the United States after the Flexner Report.

Family Practice

The American Board of Family Practice, a full-fledged specialty board, was set up in 1969 after years of promotion of the idea by the American College of General Practice. By the end of the 1970s, 367 residency programs had been established throughout the nation.[12] The residency content varied greatly among the programs, but all required at least three years of supervised hospital-based work, comprising usually a combination of internal medicine, pediatrics, psychiatry, and obstetrics and gynecology. The conspicuous omission was surgery and its subspecialties, although in most residencies training was provided on outpatient minor surgical procedures.

The first nationwide survey of general and family practitioners was made in 1977, and at that time it was found that only 13 percent had completed residency training, in order to be eligible for specialty status. There was a marked difference with age-level, however. Among practitioners under 35 years of age, the proportion who had completed family practice residencies was 50 percent, with a sharp fall-off to less than 10 percent in those over age 35. Of the national sample studied, some 30 percent were Board certified in family practice (occasionally in another field) and 70 percent were traditional general practitioners.

The age distribution of those completing residencies, of course, indicates the trends. If young medical graduates continue to be attracted to family practice as a specialty, it is likely that in time they will largely replace the traditional G.P. As of 1977, about 65 percent of family and general practitioners were engaged in private solo medical practice, 26 percent were in group practice (single-specialty or multispecialty), and the balance (9 percent) were in other special circumstances. There is a somewhat greater tendency for family and general practitioners to be located outside of metropolitan areas or in rural localities than for other physicians.

Office-based general and family practitioners have, on the average, 167.4 patient encounters per week, seeing an average of 3.38 patients per hour. This is a greater number of patients served than is served by other doctors; it explains why these generalists provide about one-third of all ambulatory visits in the nation although they constitute only 11.5 percent of physicians in office-based practice.

The general or family practitioner is the provider of primary care, *par excellence*. With the worldwide emphasis on the importance of primary health care, tabulation of primary care doctors in the United States has been subject to debate. Some analysts count pediatricians and internists as primary care doctors, although many of them engage in subspecialties—especially the majority of internists who focus on cardiology, endocrinology, nephrology, rheumatology, and so on. Some consider obstetrician-gynecologists as providers of primary care, although they obviously deal with only one organ system in women. The entire issue concerning the most suitable arrangements for primary health care in America reflects the problem of medical fragmentation through the specialties.[13] Coordination and teamwork among specialists is achieved to some extent in group practice clinics and in hospitals that have good medical staff organization. Until such teamwork is more widely achieved, the family practice of medicine provides for many patients the comprehensive scope of service that is so often required.

In developing countries, the shortage of primary health care doctors, especially in rural areas, has given rise to a variety of briefly trained "community health workers," medical assistants, or "barefoot doctors."[14] The idea of "middle-level" physician-substitutes arose in the nineteenth century in Czarist Russia, where they were called "feldshers"; these were trained even by the Soviet government long after the socialist revolution. In the mid-1960s, when the supply of physicians was deemed adequate, the output of feldshers for general primary care was reduced, and their work became restricted to ambulances, laboratories, or various first-aid stations.

In the United States, similarly, an initial response to the shortage of primary care doctors was the training of "physician assistants," from ex-medical corpsmen returning from the Vietnam War in the 1960s. Then, as discussed earlier, "nurse practitioners" were trained for the provision of primary care, with only limited supervision by doctors. While many of these new types of health personnel were deployed in rural areas and urban slums, often working alone, the discriminatory attitude to the poor, implicit in this policy, has gradually become recognized.[15] As more family practitioners (and more physicians as a whole) have been educated, the demand for both nurse practitioners and physician assistants has declined, and those already trained are now working predominantly in clinic teams, along with doctors and others.

Health Personnel for Long-Term Care

Illness in the aging person typically involves multiple diagnoses, so that this type of patient more than most others requires the skills and attitudes of a primary care physician. In the 1977 study of family and general practice, discussed above, it was found that persons over age 65—while constituting about 10 percent of the population—entailed 17 percent of the ambulatory care encounters. Aged people, of course, utilize a higher rate of ambulatory service from doctors as a whole, but the visits to general and family practitioners constituted in 1981 more than 34 percent of the visits to all physicians.

The health services required by aged and chronically ill patients in hospitals are relatively even greater.[16] In 1981, when the U.S. national population was admitted to hospitals at the rate of 160.2 cases and 1134 days per 1000 persons per year, the comparable figures for those over 65 were 396.5 admissions and 4155 days per 1000 persons per year. Beyond this are the still larger numbers of persons using nursing homes with different levels of care. In the late 1970s, some 18,000 nursing homes accommodated on the average day 1,303,100 patients, of whom 86 percent were over 65 years of age. This constituted 4.8 percent of persons over 65, but over age 85, the rate was 21.6 percent.

For all these institutionalized patients, the needs for health personnel are obviously great. Most important are nurses, and most state laws licensing nursing homes require that a registered (professional) nurse be on duty or available at all times. Very often, however, only one such fully qualified nurse is available, and the great bulk of patient care is provided by licensed vocational nurses or nursing attendants with very little formal training. This is not to overlook the fact that many middle-aged women, without formal training, learn a great deal through experience and provide effective and sensitive care for elderly patients. In better quality institutions for long-term care, the services of rehabilitation therapists and social workers are also furnished on a part-time or full-time basis.

Perhaps the greatest personnel problems concern physicians, with appropriate orientation to the care of the aged and chronically ill patient. To some extent, every general and family practitioner may have the necessary competence, but in many it is weakly developed. The same applies to the general or the subspecialized internist. Most physicians unfortunately have been found to spend less time with elderly patients and even avoid serving patients who are in nursing homes. Very few nursing homes are staffed with a full-time physician in the facility. In a nationwide survey, only 0.2 percent of all U.S. physicians considered geriatrics to be their primary or even secondary interest.

The Institute of Medicine of the National Academy of Sciences has recommended that "geriatric medicine" should be recognized as an academic subspecialty field, under the general rubric of internal medicine.[17] A few medical schools have begun to give special instruction in the field—in geriatrics or more broadly in gerontology—but the special needs of elderly patients should also be taught throughout the medical school curriculum. This need is particularly great in the teaching of psychiatry. The need should be recognized also in the training programs for all the other health professions.

REFERENCES

1. National Center for Health Statistics: Health—United States 1983. Washington, DC: GPO, 1983; 160.
2. Donabedian A, Axelrod SJ, Wyszewianski L: Medical Care Chartbook (7th ed). Ann Arbor, Mich: AUPHA Press, 1980.
3. US Department of Commerce, Bureau of the Census: Historical Statistics of the United States, Colonial Times to 1970, Part I. Washington, DC: GPO, 1976.
4. US Department of Commerce, Bureau of the Census: Statistical Abstracts of the United States: 1915, 34th Number and 1974, 95th ed. Washington, DC: GPO, 1915, 1974.
5. US Department of Commerce, Bureau of the Census: 1980 Census of Population, Vol. 2, Subject Reports. Earnings by Occupation and Education. Washington, DC: GPO, 1984.
6. US Department of Health and Human Services, Bureau of Health Professions: Source Book—Nursing Personnel. DHHS Pub. No. (HRA) 81–21, 1981.
7. National League for Nursing: NLN Nursing Data Book 1983–1984. New York: NLN Pub. No. 19–1954, 1984.
8. American Nurses' Association: Facts About Nursing 82–83, Kansas City: ANA, 1983. (*See also* US Department of Health and Human Services, Bureau of Health Professions: The Registered Nurse Population: An Overview from National Sample of Registered Nurses, November 1980. Revised November 1982. DHHS Pub. No. HRS–P–OD–83–1, 1983.)
9. Kim MJ, McFarland GK, McLane AM (Eds): Classification of Nursing Diagnosis: Proceedings of the Fifth National Congress. St. Louis: Mosby, 1984.
10. Kalisch PA, Kalisch BJ: The Advance of American Nursing. Boston: Little, Brown, 1978.
11. Aiken LH (Ed.): Nursing in the 1980's: Crises, Opportunities, Challenges. Philadelphia: Lippincott, 1982.
12. Rosenblatt RA, *et al:* The structure and content of family practice: Current status and future trends. J Fam Prac, October 1982; 15:681–722.
13. Yankauer A: Who shall deliver primary care? Am J Public Health 1980; 70:1048.
14. Jensen RT: The primary medical care worker in developing countries. Med Care Nov.–Dec. 1967; 5:382–400.
15. Roemer MI: Primary care and physician extenders in affluent countries. Int J Health Serv Fall 1977; 7:545–555.
16. Ouslander JG, Beck JC: Defining the health problems of the elderly. Ann Rev Public Health 1982, 3:55–83.
17. Institute of Medicine: Aging and Medical Education. Washington, DC: National Academy of Sciences, 1978.

Chapter **5**

Integration of Medical Care and Health Promotion

Since the mid-1970s, there has been a kind of rediscovery of prevention in the United States, Canada, and other industrialized countries, due to expanding epidemiological knowledge about factors contributing to noncommunicable chronic diseases, and to the mounting complexities and costs of medical treatment, among other things. The new emphasis on prevention in America has pushed aside the controversial issue of national health insurance (NHI), with its implication of higher governmental expenditures and more regulation.

In developing countries, where elementary environmental sanitation is still grossly deficient, the priority for prevention has long been recognized by health leaders (although not necessarily acted upon). In the United States, however, the recent tendency to counterpose prevention to medical care, heralding the value of health promotion while denigrating the wastefulness of treatment, creates a false dichotomy. In affluent industrialized countries, any sharp line between prevention and treatment is unsound. In both theory and practice, prevention and medical care reinforce each other.

This chapter will attempt to show the importance of *integrated* prevention and medical care in the health policy formulation of all countries, but especially in the modern industrialized countries. It will discuss: (1) the reasons for the recent denigration of medical care, (2) the great achievements of prevention, (3) the benefits of modern medical care, (4) the specific value of medical care for disease prevention and health promotion, and (5) the implications of this analysis for policy in national health care systems.

DENIGRATION OF MEDICAL CARE

Skepticism about the value of medical care became prominent in the mid-1970s, in large part as a reaction to the rising complexities of medical technology (both diagnostic and therapeutic) and the mounting costs of its use. In its more extreme form, this was articulated by Ivan Illich, a former priest,[1] and Rick Carlson, a lawyer.[2] Illich went so far as to claim that physicians usually did more harm than good.

A preference for "natural" over artificial methods of health service and health maintenance has been asserted by many people for years. It was reflected in the early opposition to immunizations, to the pasteurization of milk, and the chlorination of water supplies, and it is still seen in the opposition by some people to water fluoridation for reducing dental caries. Homeopathy arose in opposition to the copious use of drugs in nineteenth-century medicine, and chiropractic—acclaimed as "drugless healing"—arose in reaction to any use of drugs.[3] But when the man-made technology became more and more expensive, with sometimes uncertain evidence of benefits, the arguments against it intensified.[4]

The whole value of clinical medicine, in contrast to the importance of good living conditions, has long been forcefully questioned by public health leaders and scholars. Thomas McKeown has shown that in England the infant mortality rate and mortality from tuberculosis began their declines in the early nineteenth century, long before the discovery of the microorganisms that caused these deaths and the development of public health and medical strategies to combat them.[5] In 1790, Johann Peter Franck had spoken of "the people's misery" or poverty as the "mother of diseases."[6] René Sand, the great Belgian scholar of social medicine, wrote in 1936 of how the achievements of public health dwarfed those of individual physicians.[7] In 1944, C.-E. A. Winslow, reacting to extravagant claims of the American Medical Association, showed that the great reduction in American death rates between 1900 and 1940 was "due predominantly to public health programs rather than clinical medicine."[8]

In spite of the modest past accomplishments of medical treatment, relative to those attributable to improved living standards and public health programs, the rising expenditures for medical care have become increasingly conspicuous. In the United States, where such data have been collected for over 50 years, national expenditures for all health purposes rose from \$3.6 billion in 1929 to \$247.2 billion in 1980, an escalation from 3.5 percent of the gross national product (GNP) to 9.4 percent.[9] The slope of the expenditure curve became especially steep after 1950. Furthermore, about 92 percent of this expenditure was for medical care, and hardly 3 percent for organized public health activities.

By 1970, the costs of medical care were rising so rapidly that proposals for national health insurance (NHI), quiescent since 1950, arose from many quarters.[10] But other issues took precedence, and by the time of the Carter Administration, 1976–1980, the NHI issue receded before charges that it was "too expensive." Raising the banner of prevention, therefore, coincided very nicely with the retreat from NHI; presumably, it was both cheaper and better. Even the conservative medical establishment joined in the rediscovery of prevention. Why should the nation's whole system of medical care be assaulted, when social improvements to promote health would be less costly and more effective? In the words of a leading U.S. medical spokesman in 1976:

> It is one of the great and sobering truths of our profession that modern health care probably has less impact on the health of the population than economic status, education, housing, nutrition, and sanitation . . . yet knowing that, I think we have fostered the idea that abundant, readily available, high quality health care would be some kind of panacea for the ills of society and the individual. That is a fiction, a hoax . . .[11]

Public action for improving economic access to personal medical care, one would infer, was really not so important.

Within the enormous U.S. expenditures for medical care, the largest and also the most rapidly growing segment was for patient care in hospitals. In 1950, hospitals had absorbed 30.4 percent of the total spending, rising to 40.3 percent in 1980. If nursing home costs are added, institutional expenditures amounted to 48.7 percent of the total in 1980, not including the services of doctors to bed patients.[9] One can appreciate why so much of the mounting skepticism about medical care has been focused on hospitals, where high costs and high technology come together.

Hospitals are also the places where doctors perform surgery, for much of which the justification is being questioned. Several studies have shown that rates of surgical operations vary directly with the local ratio of surgeons to a population, more than with evidence of health need.[12, 13] When the doctor's financial incentives are changed from fee-for-service to salary, as in health maintenance organizations (HMOs), the rates of elective surgery invariably decline; yet the predominant evidence indicates that the quality of care in HMOs and the health record of HMO members are superior to these indicators in the private medical market.[14] High costs aggravate the discontent of patients not cured by surgical intervention; in back of most of the numerous malpractice suits in America, one nearly always finds an angry patient.[15]

In developing countries, the imbalance of health resource allocations for hospitals, in contrast to public health programs, is particularly striking.[16] Yet in these countries the enormous burden of preventable disease should favor the highest priorities for prevention and primary care. This policy is constantly promoted by the World Health Organization.[17] And although it is all too seldom followed, the WHO emphases on "appropriate technology," "primary health care," and "community participation" underscore the worldwide advocacy of prevention in preference to medical care.

ACHIEVEMENTS OF PREVENTION

The massive achievements of improved environmental sanitation and communicable disease control in extending life expectancy in industrialized countries are well known. Reductions in the mortality of infants and small children have been most important, but the near-conquest of tuberculosis in the industrialized countries has contributed substantially to lower mortality in the adult years. The burden of physical disability was greatly reduced by development of immunization against poliomyelitis in 1954. Greater knowledge of nutrition, along with school feeding programs, social insurance pensions, and public assistance for the poor, have almost eliminated the diseases of hunger in the industrialized countries.

In the place of death and disability from infectious disease, the major problems in the developed countries became the chronic noncommunicable disorders.[18] The potentialities of preventing these diseases are increasingly appreciated. The periodic health examination has adjusted itself to the demographic distribution of disease in populations.[19] Mass examinations for syphilis and tuberculosis have been supplemented by blood glucose determinations for diabetes, ocular tonometry for glaucoma, Papanicalaou smears for cervical cancer, and so on. In America, combinations of these tests in "multiphasic screening" programs became a strategy for prevention.[20] Even though the general concept has not been accepted universally,[21] the value of early disease detection has been demonstrated for various disorders.

In the 1950s, the relationship of fat consumption to arteriosclerosis and coronary artery disease was shown by Ancel Keys and others.[22] The exact mechanisms are still under study and debate, but there has developed a wide consensus that saturated fats—along with lack of exercise, cigarette smoking, and stress—are "risk factors" in the genesis of cardiovascular disease. As early as 1938, Raymond Pearl reported on the negative statistical relationship between smoking and longevity,[23] and in the early 1950s Richard Doll produced convincing evidence of the causal role of tobacco in lung cancer.[24] The pathogenic role of alcohol consumption in cirrhosis of the liver had long been known, and its contribution to serious automobile accidents has become gradually more prominent.

These and other epidemiological findings provide increasingly firm foundations to a strategy for preventing the major causes of death in most industrialized countries. In 1965, Lester Breslow and colleagues began their longitudinal studies of some 7000 adults in one California county, showing the relationship of "health habits" (dietary practices, smoking, drinking, sleeping, etc.) to mortality.[25] In 1974, the Annual Report of the Canadian Minister of National Health and Welfare, Marc Lalonde, attracted worldwide attention in calling for changes in human behavior as the heart of a "new perspective" for improving health.[26] By the late 1970s, everyone was speaking of the importance of "lifestyle" for good health. The U.S. Surgeon General summarized the accumulated knowledge in a 1979 Report on Health Promotion and Disease Prevention.[27]

The ecology movement of the 1960s gave further impetus to the rediscovery of prevention. Increasing air pollution in the large cities, stream pollution from industrial wastes, the international issues of nuclear bomb tests and radioactive fallout—all these problems led to a fresh appreciation of the importance of a clean environment.[28] The anti-war movement of the 1960s reinforced the demands for a society free from man-made violence and the many abuses of nature by modern civilization.

By the 1980s, the momentum for an active social policy of prevention and positive health promotion was very strong. Joggers were everywhere, and exercise of all kinds was promoted for the sedentary city dweller. Cigarette packages were required by law in some 40 countries to warn of the grave dangers of smoking.[29] Fat preparations in the market emphasized their composition of "unsaturated" lipids and absence of cholesterol. Laws were passed to require seat belts in automobiles, and some countries made it an offense for riders not to use them.

In the late 1970s and early 1980s, the strategies for prevention of chronic noncommunicable disease began to show an effect. While the precise explanations were elusive, certain types of cancer—such as cervical in women and stomach cancer in both sexes—had been definitely declining. When the mortality rate from heart disease in the United States was examined on an age-adjusted basis, it was found that after steady escalation it had begun to decline from 308 per 100,000 in 1950 to 208 in 1978.[9] Death rates from lung cancer, associated with smoking, continued to rise, but there was much evidence that this lethal practice was lessening, especially in adult males.

How much of the impressive decline in U.S. cardiac mortality was due to improved medical care, however, and how much to the several preventive strategies is not clear. In the 1950s and perhaps the early 1960s, the preventive policies were not widespread, and advances in clinical cardiology may well deserve the major credit. By the late 1960s and the 1970s, perhaps preventive behavior played the greater part. Comparison with trends in the Soviet Union suggest this inference. Between 1964 and 1975 there was an 18 percent increase in Soviet cardiac death rates,[30] with a concomitant increase in the consumption of animal fats and of tobacco in the USSR. During this same period, U.S. consumption of these products declined.

Even U.S. mortality from accidents declined from 58 per 100,000 in 1950 to 44 in 1978, influenced perhaps by the global oil crisis, automobile seat belts, and lower highway speed limits. The prevalence of dental caries also declined in the 1970s, presumably as a result of fluoridation of water supplies and other forms of fluoride intake.[31] Thus the achievements of prevention, quite outside the sphere of communicable diseases, were very impressive indeed.

BENEFITS OF MEDICAL CARE

The demonstrable achievements of prevention, combined with the continued escalation of the costs of therapy, led naturally to political and social pressures for containment of the rising costs of medical care,[32] creating an artificial dichotomy between prevention (with high value and low cost) and treatment (with low value and high cost). Unfortunately, such a dichotomy not only overlooks the many benefits derived from medical care, but also ignores the great value of the medical care process as a major channel for the delivery of preventive health service.

The great extensions of U.S. life expectancy at birth—from 47.3 years in 1900 to 73.3 years in 1978—has been due mainly to reduction in the mortality rate of infants and small children. Mortality in the first year of life is widely recognized to reflect living conditions, but these exert their influence principally *after* the neonatal period (the first 28 days of life). Neonatal death rates in the United States have declined from about 45 per 1000 live births in 1915 to 9.5 per 1000 in 1978,[33] due in large part to improved handling of the childbirth process, including delivery of newborns in hospitals—a component of medical care. The abrupt decline in U.S. infant mortality between 1965 (24.7 per 1000 live births) and 1975 (16.1 per 1000) was probably not merely coincidental with the Medicaid program that financed medical care for the babies of poor families in those years.

At the other end of the life scale, at age 65, to what extent can one attribute the extension in life expectancy to preventive services or to lifestyle? Before 1960, the lifestyle strategy for prevention was hardly significant, yet United States life expectancy in 1900 at age 65 was 11.9 additional years; by 1960, it was 14.3 additional years,[9] an increase of 20.2 percent, surely a benefit predominantly of medical care. By 1978, life expectancy at age 65 was extended an additional 2.0 years to 16.3 years. During this 18-year period (1960–1978), preventive strategies may have been mainly responsible for the extra longevity, but the medical treatment of heart disease, cancer, diabetes, pneumonia, and other diseases of old age must also have made a substantial contribution. For the years 1965–1975, a national conference, studying the decline in U.S. cardiac mortality, could not decide how much was attributable to changes in lifestyle and how much to improved medical care.[34]

Rather striking evidence of the influence of access to medical care on the mortality rates of the aged is shown in age-specific data comparing the United States and Canada.[35] In 1966–1967, the age-adjusted death rate of all American women was 5.7 per 1000, compared with 5.1 per 1000 in Canada; the Canadian record was better than that of the United States for all age groups. In 1966, it will be recalled, the U.S.

Medicare and Medicaid programs went into effect, making medical service financially accessible to virtually all Americans 65 years of age and older. Financially accessible care was available to all Canadians in 1966. A decade later, in 1976–1977, the age-specific mortality rates of both populations had declined; those of U.S. women were still higher than those of Canadian women at all specific age levels except 65-and-over. In this age group, which in the United States had been entitled to socially financed medical care for a decade, the relationship reversed and the U.S. mortality rate became lower than that of Canada (36.0 vs. 37.5 per 1000, respectively). The dynamics were less dramatic for elderly males, but in the same general direction.

When mortality rates are reduced, whether by prevention or medical care or both, one should not expect a commensurate reduction in morbidity or disability. Each additional day or year that a person stays alive, he becomes part of the population at risk for all causes of disease and injury. This simple truth is often overlooked, and yet it accounts for the rising rates of disability over time, when mortality rates are declining. The U.S. National Health Survey found that the rate of "restricted-activity days," age-adjusted, rose from 17.0 per person per year in 1974 to 18.5 in 1979.[9] For acute conditions, the incidence rose from 204 per 1000 persons per year in 1970 to 222 in 1979. These trends apply to both the young (under age 17) and the elderly (over age 65), examined separately. Prevention, therefore, does not reduce the need for medical care in the long run.

Skeptics may say that adding years to life after age 65 tells us nothing about the quality of life in those extra years. A crucial benefit of medical care, however, is precisely its impact on the quality of life—that is, on the ability of the patient to be free from symptoms, to function socially, and to be happy.

Walsh McDermott, referring to the "personal encounter physician system" in contrast to the "public health system,"[36] speaks of the thousands of patients with serious heart disease who are not only kept alive, but are enabled to work and function socially by skillful medical care; patients with degenerated hip joints who are enabled to walk again; diabetics, who cannot be cured, but can be kept alive and fully effective for decades. Tracing the trend of U.S. age-adjusted death rates for all causes, McDermott points to the steady decline from 1900 to 1937, then the abruptly steeper downward slope for the next 20 years. During those 20 years, there was no major change in lifestyle, no major new preventive strategy, but the sulfa drugs appeared in 1937 and penicillin in 1945. Administration of these drugs, which constitutes medical care, was doubtless responsible for saving the lives of thousands of patients with pneumonia, septicemia, osteomyelitis, and other bacterial infections that had not been prevented.

Medical care is the principal control strategy for hypertension, one of the major risk factors in cardiovascular disease and cerebrovascular accidents; medications do not cure the disease but control it so that the patient stays well. Glaucoma, one of the major causes of blindness in the industrialized countries, is treated with eye medication that does not cure the disease, but reduces intra-ocular pressure so that vision does not deteriorate. Pharmaceutical control of serious psychoses—schizophrenia and manic-depressive psychosis—has reduced the occupancy of mental hospitals enormously and has enabled thousands of mental patients to live in their home communities.[37] Psychopharmaceutical therapy has also greatly reduced disability from depressive disorders—probably the commonest of all psychoneurotic afflictions.

The quality of life is admittedly difficult to measure, but there is no doubt that medical care can improve it to some extent in virtually all diseases. Much gynecological surgery may be unjustified, but hysterectomies eliminate distressing symptoms in millions of women. The patient with rheumatoid arthritis may not be curable, but he/she can be enabled to live comfortably and to avoid getting permanent deformities. The life-saving value of emergency medical care for serious injuries is dramatized daily. The beneficial effects of primary medical care, for patients with various chronic disorders, have been quantified in terms of simple aspects of behavior, such as improvements in locomotion, sleeping, eating, and other activities of daily life.[38] Finally, one must not ignore the emotional value of medical reassurance, when this is feasible.

Perhaps the most convincing evidence of the benefits of medical care has been provided by Jack Hadley's recent analysis of mortality rates in 400 U.S. counties. Using demographic data from the 1970 Census and medical care utilization data drawn from other sources (but not the customary physician–population ratio), he concludes:

> The principal finding of this study is that medical care has a negative and statistically significant impact on mortality rates. This implies that health is better when medical care use is higher. After controlling for other

factors, such as income, education, marital status, work experience, cigarette consumption, and disability, cohorts with greater estimated use of medical care appear to have lower mortality rates (for all causes of death). . . . A 10 percent increase in medical care expenditures per capita is estimated to reduce mortality rates by between 1.23 percent (elderly white males) and 2.04 percent (black female infants), with an average reduction of 1.57 percent.[39]

It would seem reasonable to infer that this reduction in mortality rates, associated with medical care, implies also a corresponding improvement in the quality of living during the additional duration of life achieved.

The economic benefits of medical care should not be overlooked. Early and effective treatment of most diseases can reduce not only days of disability but also days lost from work and the subsequent drains on disability insurance funds. Rehabilitative care has converted many invalids from welfare clients to workers who pay taxes.

VALUE OF MEDICAL CARE FOR PREVENTION

The linkage between prevention and treatment was emphasized years ago when Hugh Leavell and Gurney Clark spoke of four "levels of prevention:" (1) health promotion, (2) protection against specific disorders, (3) early disease detection with prompt treatment, and (4) limitation of disability.[40] The first level is exemplified by good nutrition, the second by immunizations, the third by screening programs, and the fourth by rehabilitation. It would seem that many have still not understood this basic concept.

When the patient with chest pains is advised by the doctor to lose weight, exercise moderately, sleep more, and stop smoking, how much preventive service is he getting and how much medical care? When a Pap smear reveals an early cervical cancer, and prompt surgery saves the woman's life, is this prevention or medical care? The answer, of course, is "both." The competent, conscientious physician almost inevitably gives preventive service when he renders medical care.

The patient seeking help for an ailment presents the opportunity for appropriate personal preventive service. A thoughtful word from the doctor about not smoking is bound to be more effective than printed warnings on a thousand packs of cigarettes. Education on prudent changes in behavior can be focused on the varying needs of each individual. But such prevention depends on access to medical care when needed. In developing countries, it was learned long ago that provision of treatment for people's ailments is the surest way to attract them to the health centers or health posts, where preventive services are offered.[41]

In day-to-day medical care by private practitioners, however, the opportunities for prevention are only rarely exploited. The average physician is oriented to the treatment of disease, the relief of his/her patient's symptoms. Many health insurance programs, in fact, specifically exclude payment for preventive services, since they are not an "unpredictable risk." As John Freymann has pointed out, the average doctor tends to associate prevention with government and mass collective actions; he sees his role as personal and curative.[42] But this perception of the doctor's role is not inevitable. A rationally planned health care system could achieve an integration of prevention and medical care that would strengthen the effectiveness of both.

First of all, health service, both therapeutic and preventive, must be accessible to everyone. Access requires more than financial support, although such support is essential. In the majority of industrialized countries, this economic foundation has been provided through national health insurance (NHI) or equivalent public revenue programs. Many of these programs require stronger funding, improved relationships with providers, greater scope of benefits, and other improvements.[43] In the United States, where NHI protection applies only to the aged—and far from completely for them—the need for public action to assure universal access to comprehensive health services is much greater. Judging by the experience of other nations, the very conversion of health care costs into a social responsibility sets in motion forces for achieving greater efficiency and effectiveness in the patterns of organization of health services.[44]

But more than money is needed to achieve integration of prevention and treatment. Physicians and other health personnel must be taught to appreciate the importance of prevention in their relationship with every patient. Education in medicine and allied fields would require substantial revision to heighten the graduate's sensitivity, not only to health promotion and prevention, but also to the entire social and environmental setting that influences health. Continuing education should attempt to maintain this knowledge and attitude as regularly as it is concerned with advances in biomedical science.

Health facilities would also require substantial modification. If hospitals are to offer integrated care, they must be designed to furnish personal preventive service to both outpatients and inpatients, to have equipment for large-scale screening tests, to offer continuing health education to groups large and small. Ambulatory care centers should be accessible in every urban and rural area, as the major settings for integrated delivery of preventive and treatment services.

The integration of prevention and medical care involves more than health service. It calls for concern by health authorities with every person's employment, housing, nutrition, community relationships, and all the other influences on health—the perspective that WHO defines as "intersectoral cooperation." It means devoting attention to conditions in the child's school and the worker's factory or farm. Organizationally, such policies require coordination between health and other public authorities at every political level.

Within the health sector, in most countries, the organizational cleavages leading to inequalities and inequities are very great. Within government, there is needless fragmentation in the care of various population groups and disorders. Most serious is the large distinction between publicly sponsored and private-market health services. Insofar as health care is a private market commodity, its distribution is obviously based on personal wealth more than health need. If prevention and medical care are to be effectively integrated, deliberate strategies must build the whole framework of the health care system on principles of equity.

The administration and regulation of the health care system would have to be much more unified than it is in the pluralistic setting of the United States. This does not mean total centralization. Wide variations in local program implementation should be feasible and encouraged, under a broad national health policy. A regulatory process should be built into the system structure, instead of involving policing from the outside.

At the point of health service delivery, the changes from present patterns would be most important. There would be no reason for special "well-baby clinics" to give preventive service, while private doctors or hospital outpatient departments treated the sick child. Teams of health personnel working in health centers should be the norm for both types of service.

Every person should have a primary care doctor who serves as the gateway and guide to the whole health care system. As more is learned about the "epidemiology of health," more information, advice, and guidance could be provided to patients.[45] Local health centers would have to be backed up by hospitals which must, in turn, be appropriately linked to other hospitals in a regional framework. For reasons of both economy and quality, there would have to be efficient logistics for the distribution of drugs and supplies.

With respect to environmental sanitation, it is worth recalling that in the early nineteenth century there were many accounts of poor health among Americans, particularly women and children. The common answer to the problem "was found not in public health measures but in encouraging the practice of personal hygiene. . . . In the main, the necessity of more exercise and suitable outdoor pastimes was emphasized."[46] It was only in the later nineteenth and early twentieth centuries that the importance of proper sanitation, good nutrition, and decent housing was appreciated.

Today also we must take care that we are not misled into thinking that a sound lifestyle is the main key to good health and should be sought solely through behavioral modification. For example, in 1976, John Knowles, then President of the Rockefeller Foundation, wrote: "The next major advances in the health of the American people will result from the assumption of individual responsibility for one's own health."[47] The lifestyle argument has been epitomized as "blaming the victim," which may be stretching the point too far, but it is obviously crucial to identify the *social* causes of unhygienic behavior and do something about them.[48] The most obvious contradiction is seen in the current psychological strategies to discourage smoking, while at the same time permitting massive cigarette advertising and subsidizing tobacco farmers.

Integrated prevention and medical care are bound to be less expensive than separate arrangements, if only because of economies of scale and savings on transportation. But most important is the practical convenience for people, the administrative efficiency, and the greater community impact of providing preventive and treatment services at the same local facilities, often at the same time.[49] The customary separation of prevention and medical care in the free market countries has been due to political, not managerial, considerations.

In summary, a health policy emphasizing prevention is sound in all types of countries, but such a policy should not be regarded as antagonistic to a national program of medical care for all. Access to treatment enhances the opportunities for prevention in countless ways. Moreover, once the major infectious diseases and malnutrition are eliminated, medical care has substantial value in extending lives and improving the quality of life. A health care system that makes integrated preventive/ therapeutic health service accessible to everyone—financially, geographically, and psychologically—would have the greatest human and economic value.

REFERENCES

1. Illich I: Medical Nemesis: The Expropriation of Health. New York: Random House, 1975.
2. Carlson R: The End of Medicine. New York: Wiley, 1975.
3. Reed LS: The Healing Cults. Chicago: University of Chicago Press, 1932.
4. Fuchs V: Who Shall Live? New York: Basic Books, 1974.
5. McKeown T: The Role of Medicine: Dream, Mirage, or Nemesis. London: Nuffield Provincial Hospitals Trust, 1976.
6. Sigerist HE: Landmarks in the History of Hygiene. London: Oxford University Press, 1956; 47–63.
7. Sand R: Health and Human Progress. New York: Macmillan, 1936.
8. Winslow C-EA: Who killed cock robin? Am J Public Health 1944; 34:658–659.
9. National Center for Health Statistics: Health—United States 1981. DHHS Pub. No. PHS 82–1232. Washington, DC: GPO, 1982.
10. US Social Security Administration: National Health Insurance Proposal. HEW Pub. No. SSA 76–11920. Washington, DC: GPO, 1976.
11. Cooper T: (US Assistant Secretary for Health) quoted in report of The National Leadership Conference on America's Health Policy. Washington, DC, April 29–30, 1976.
12. Bunker JP, Wennberg JE: Operation rates, mortality statistics, and the quality of life. N Engl J Med 1973; 289:1249–1251.
13. Lewis CE: Variations in the incidence of surgery. N Engl J Med 1969; 291:880–884.
14. Luft JE: Health Maintenance Organizations: Dimensions of Performance. New York: Wiley, 1981.
15. Schwartz DH: Societal Responsibility for Malpractice. Health and Society, Milbank Mem Fund Q Fall 1976; 54:469–488.
16. Abel-Smith B. Leiserson A: Poverty, Development, and Health Policy. Geneva: World Health Organization, 1978; 67.
17. World Health Organization: Formulating Strategies for Health for All by the Year 2000. Geneva: WHO, 1979.
18. World Health Organization: Sixth Report on the World Health Situation. 1973–1977. Part I: Global analysis. Geneva: WHO, 1980; 37–50.
19. Roemer MI: A program of preventive medicine for the individual. Milbank Mem Fund Q 1945; 23:209–226.

20. Gelman AC: Multiphasic Health Testing Systems: Reviews and Annotations. Washington, DC: National Center for Health Services Research and Development, March 1971.
21. McKeown T. *et al:* Screening in Medical Care: Reviewing the Evidence. London: Oxford University Press, 1968.
22. Keys A: Prediction and possible prevention of coronary disease. Am J Public Health 1953; 3:1399–1407.
23. Pearl R: Smoking and longevity. Science 1938; 87:(2253):216–217.
24. Doll R, Hill B: Study of aetiology of cancer of the lung. Br Med J 1952; 2:1271–1286.
25. Belloc NB, Breslow L: Relationship of physical health status and health practices. Prev Med 1972; 1:409–421.
26. Lalonde M: A New Perspective on the Health of Canadians: A Working Document. Ottawa: Health and Welfare Canada, April 1974.
27. US Public Health Service: Healthy People: The Surgeon-General's Report on Health Promotion and Disease Prevention. Washington, DC: GPO, 1979.
28. Whittenberger JL: The physical and chemical environment. *In:* Clark DW, MacMahon B: Preventive Medicine. Boston: Little, Brown, 1967; 623–642.
29. Roemer R: Legislative Action to Combat the World Smoking Epidemic. Geneva: World Health Organization, 1982.
30. Cooper R, Schatzkin A: Recent trends in coronary risk factors in the USSR. Am J Public Health 1982; 72:431–440.
31. Knutson JW: Water fluoridation after 25 years. J Am Dent Assoc 1970; 80:765.
32. Schweitzer SO (Ed): Policies for the containment of health care costs and expenditures. DHEW Pub. No. NIH 78–184. Washington, DC: Department of Health, Education and Welfare, 1978.
33. Donabedian A, Axelrod SJ, Wyszewianski L: Medical Care Chart Book—Seventh Ed. Ann Arbor, Mich.: Health Administration Press, 1980.
34. US Public Health Service. Proceedings of the Conference on the Decline in Coronary Heart Disease Mortality. DHEW Pub. No. (NIH)79–1610. Washington, DC: GPO, 1979.
35. Anon: Mortality in the United States, Canada, and Western Europe. Metropolitan Life Insurance Company Statistical Bulletin 1981; 62(4):10–13.
36. McDermott W: Medicine: The Public Good and One's Own. World Health Forum 1979; 1:125–234.
37. Serban G (Ed): New Trend of Psychiatry in the Community. Cambridge, MA: Ballinger, 1977.
38. McDowell I, Martini CJM: Problems and new directions in the evaluation of primary care. Int J Epidemiol 1976; 5:247–250.
39. Hadley J: More Medical Care, Better Health? Washington, DC: Urban Institute Press, 1982; 8.
40. Leavell HR, Clark EG: Textbook of Preventive Medicine. New York: McGraw-Hill, 1953; 7–27.
41. Roemer MI: Evaluation of Community Health Centers. Geneva: World Health Organization (Public Health Paper No. 48), 1973.

42. Freymann JG: Medicine's great schism: prevention vs. cure: an historical interpretation. Med Care 1975; 13:525–536.
43. Fulcher D: Medical Care Systems: Public and Private Health Coverage in Selected Industrial Countries. Geneva: International Labor Office, 1974.
44. Roemer MI: From health insurance to health care systems—an international view. *In:* Social Medicine: The Advance of Organized Health Services in America. New York: Springer, 1978; 530–543.
45. Terris M: Approaches to an epidemiology of health. Am J Public Health 1975; 65:1037–1045.
46. Kramer HD: The beginnings of the public health movement in the United States. Bull Hist Med 1947; 21:352–376.
47. Knowles JS (Ed): Doing Better and Feeling Worse: Health in the United States. New York: WW Norton, 1977.
48. Crawford R: You are dangerous to your health: the ideology and politics of victim blaming. J Health Serv 1977; 7:663–680.
49. Yankauer A: The ups and downs of prevention (editorial). J Public Health 1981; 71:6–9.

Chapter **6**

Free Market Dynamics and Health Care Policy

In recent years it has become increasingly fashionable to attribute the many serious problems of the American health care system to "excessive government regulation." It is argued that a deliberate return to the classical entrepreneurial model of free trade and competition would solve or greatly reduce our problems of spiraling health care costs and inaccessibility of needed services. From this viewpoint, there follow many political actions to minimize the entire role of government—with respect to both regulation and planning—and to enhance the private sector in health care.[1] Under the Reagan Administration, such strategies have become explicitly dominant.

INTRODUCTION: THE BASIC ISSUE

The question of whether free trade with competition, or social planning with regulation, is the most effective mechanism for governance of the health care system has very complex ramifications. Comprehensive analysis of these issues would require a lengthy book. In this chapter we consider only the major reasons why a policy of greater free trade and lesser public regulation of health services would not reduce but would increase the problems of the U.S. health care system.

The current health care systems in the United States and other capitalist nations have survived to the present day only because they have been continuously modified by planning and regulation. Without those modifications, the effects of free market dynamics in the health care sector would have been so disastrous, so unacceptable politically, that these systems would have collapsed long ago and been replaced by completely planned and regulated health care systems. In order to solve the still persistent health care problems—involving costs, accessibility, quality, and other features—America requires not greater free trade and competition, but rather much more planning and regulation.

To understand why free trade seldom leads to a balanced market structure, resulting in efficient allocation of resources, one may identify at least five necessary conditions for achievement of that outcome:[2]

1. *Many buyers and sellers freely interacting.* If there are few sellers, as often characterizes the health sector, competition can hardly operate.

2. *No substantial economies of scale.* If such economies are possible, a competitive solution is not efficient. It is often more efficient to have one large producer (a "natural monopoly") than many small ones. Price and quality, however, must then be regulated to protect consumers, in place of competition.

3. *Low transaction costs.* If arranging the purchase of a commodity or service is, itself, a complex transaction, then the use of the market can be very costly and inefficient. The commonest solution in industry is the firm, which avoids these costs by internal planning and authority. The hospital is an obvious analogue.

4. *Adequate information.* If buyers are to exercise reasonable choices in a market of competing sellers, they must have knowledge about the product being sold. Advertising is intended theoretically to enlighten consumers on the merits of various competing products (although it has been found necessary to regulate to reduce biased or misleading information). Without clear and reliable information, how can "consumer sovereignty" be exercised to lead to selections of the "best" product?

5. *Absence of externalities.* A transaction entails "externalities" if people beyond the buyer and seller are directly affected by it. (With significant externalities, even pure competitive markets are seldom efficient.) Immunization is an obvious example; if one person is not immunized, many others may be harmed. Even if all the other conditions necessary for a competitive equilibrium hold, with significant externalities it will not be efficient.

These five conditions are not the only ones necessary for static efficiency of a competitive market, but they are sufficient to show the inapplicability of the concept to the health sector. What, in fact, are the workings of free trade and competition in the medical market? To what extent do the operations of the market result in either the long run or the short run, in "quality control, price-setting, and resource allocation" that is "desirable" or optimal for achieving the best results for the individual and for society? What is the empirical evidence on the consequences of the free trade and competition model in the health sector?

The harmful effects of a social or socioeconomic idea can be reflected in two ways: first, by identification of actions taken by society to reduce those effects, and second, by recognition of problems that persist and have not yet been fully corrected. Below we offer evidence of the first type: adjustments found necessary to compensate for the ill effects of the free market, with respect to each of the above five conditions.

ADJUSTMENTS FOR THE ILL EFFECTS OF FREE TRADE AND COMPETITION

One might offer scores of examples of social programs launched to intervene in the free market, insofar as its normal operations have yielded significant social problems. Many of these problems are perceived as failures to achieve social justice, or more specifically equitable response to the personal health needs of people. Some of the problems, as we will see, relate to economic waste; still others involve explicit harm to people.

Exposition of these social adjustments may be offered in accordance with the five conditions necessary for the effective operation of a free competitive market, as explained earlier.

The Need for Many Buyers and Sellers Freely Interacting

The ordinary medical care process is hardly conducive to comparative shopping by patients among many sellers of medical care. An essential requirement for effective doctor–patient relationships is long-term continuity in the linkage of the patient with a particular doctor; the very act of consulting another physician jeopardizes this relationship. Yet the initial choice of a doctor is often based on happenstances such as geographic location or a chance recommendation.

Little has been done deliberately to assure free interaction of many buyers and sellers of primary health care. An unplanned or spontaneous social adjustment, however, has been the great expansion of hospital "emergency" services, in response to the difficulties of patient access to ordinary primary care.[3] In effect, the spiraling utilization of hospital emergency departments for non-urgent primary care has been an adjustment to the lack of adequate numbers of primary care doctors in American communities.

Perhaps a more deliberate adjustment to the sparsity of sellers of primary medical care has been the U.S. movement of the 1960s and 1970s to train substitutes for the general practitioner, in the form of physician assistants and nurse practitioners. It is noteworthy that other affluent nations with adequate supplies of generalists have not employed such a strategy.[4] Many types of federally subsidized community health centers in poverty areas have been another American adjustment.

With respect to secondary care, specifically surgical operations, intervention to permit comparisons between sellers has been deliberate. Health insurance plans have introduced procedures for "second surgical opinions"—not to determine the lowest price bid, but to permit the patient to decide whether the surgery is truly necessary in the first place.[5] Yet even this process has been opposed by medical societies as "interference in the doctor–patient relationship."

No Substantial Economies of Scale

The social adjustments induced by the clear existence of economies of scale and the associated "natural monopolies" have been numerous.

After development of the Salk vaccine against poliomyelitis, the restricted licensing of a few large pharmaceutical firms to produce the vaccine was done in obvious recognition of the economies, as well as quality controls, in such restriction of competition. The same policy is pursued with respect to production of all vaccines in many capitalist countries, not to mention the socialist countries.

In organized health care settings, the irrationality of the competitive free market model has long been evident. Hospitals, for example, continue to make exclusive contracts with radiologists and pathologists, even though this bars competition in these specialties.[6] Without such contracts, hospital care would be less efficient and even more expensive than it is. The same basic concept of structured "closed staff" hospitals has been found to promote efficiency and quality for *all* specialty services in general hospitals throughout most of the industrialized world (capitalist and socialist).[7]

In normal comprehensive health planning, the implementation of "certificate of need" legislation to authorize new hospital construction is an obvious recognition of the value of restricting competition due to the benefits of natural monopoly.[8] Quite aside from the wastefulness of superfluous hospital beds generating unjustified utilization (see below), multiple small facilities in a community are more costly and less effective than a larger integrated facility. Similar policies govern the authorization of new pharmacies in an area, even in an entrepreneurial nation like Belgium.[9]

Low Transaction Costs

The bewildering complexities of the medical care system have induced all sorts of adjustments to the high costs of the whole transaction process.

Group medical practice is one such adjustment.[10] Over the last 40 years it has grown rapidly, as an adjustment to the complexities caused for the patient by specialization in medicine, and in spite of its reduction of competition. Thus, a reduced choice of specialists is traded off for the benefits of professional teamwork and greater convenience for the patient. The elaborate integrated mechanism of the general hospital is also, of course, an adjustment to the economic and logistical monstrosity that would result if each of the hospital's hundreds of services were to be sold as a separate market transaction.

The operations of virtually all programs of organized health care delivery are further demonstrations of the high cost and inefficiencies of multiple separate transactions. This may be illustrated by governmental health programs from the magnitude of the Veterans Administration 175-hospital network down to a Health Department prenatal clinic in one small town.

Consider the transaction costs involved in the rehabilitation of a patient with a serious disability. His needs for physician services, drugs, hospitalization, physical and occupational therapy, perhaps prosthetic appliances, occupational retraining, job placement, and much more are bewildering. The process is so complex that highly directive vocational rehabilitation programs have had to be organized in all states, under which "vocational rehabilitation counselors" cut through the complexities and make decisions for the patient, rejecting the competitive process with its high transaction costs.

Adequate Information

The deficiencies of information available to the consumer are perhaps the most widespread obstacles to the efficient operation of a free health care market. A catalogue of all the social adjustments stimulated to cope with this problem would be very lengthy, indeed, and only a few can be cited.

Free competition gave rise to countless numbers and types of unqualified practitioners, particularly with the growth of cities in nineteenth-century Europe and America. How could the average consumer be expected to distinguish the knowledgeable physician from the imposter? Licensure in medicine (and later other professions) was the solution adopted throughout the world, even though it clearly reduced competition.[11] Such restriction of the free market was preferable to the tragic consequences of treatment by charlatans.

But even licensure has been an imperfect solution in the United States, as state legislatures, clinging to free market concepts, have licensed chiropractors in almost every state; this is not merely to treat vertebral disorders (for which there may be limited justification), but to handle every type of disease.[12] Moreover, medical licensure laws have been widely misused, to protect the "competitive position" of existing practitioners rather than to safeguard consumers. Yet no state has been willing to risk the disasters that might follow from revoking licensure legislation. Instead, licensure boards are being reconstituted to include consumers as spokesmen for the public interest.[13]

Some have looked upon professional licensure and similar forms of regulation as a strategy for prohibiting innovation that might be sound. They point to the long history of opposition to new ideas by orthodox medicine—opposition to smallpox vaccination, to the infectious cause of "childbed fever," and even to the pasteurization of milk.[14] The negative American attitudes today about the use of trained midwives for normal obstetrical deliveries or of New Zealand-type "dental nurses" for the care of children are put in the same class. But the latter types of health personnel are, in fact, productively used in dozens of countries. Their nonacceptance in the United States is not caused by regulation but by the political effectiveness of the medical and dental professions in suppressing competition. When and if public pressures are mounted to change the licensure laws, these reasonable types of health personnel will be licensed in the United States, as they are elsewhere.

The countless tragedies from misinformation—often deliberately false claims—about drugs make a long and distressing saga. In the United States at the end of the nineteenth century, the unfettered free market was particularly adventurist; among other things, drugs were manufactured, labeled, and sold with complete abandon. The result was enormous deception of people by grossly false claims on packaged medications, with resultant waste of millions of dollars and doubtless thousands of lives. In response, the U.S. Congress passed the first Food and Drug Control Act in 1906, greatly restricting the free market in drug production and sales. It took additional tragedies in 1939 (scores of infant deaths from a lethal "elixir" of sulfanilamide) and in 1962 (hundreds of limbless babies born to mothers taking thalidomide) to bring further tightening of drug control legislation against the abuses of competitive free enterprise in the U.S. pharmaceutical industry.[15]

The workings of hospitals have long been far too complex to be evaluated by the average patient, even by the average community physician. Many facilities lacked proper laboratories, surgical equipment, or nursing staffs, but how was the outsider to know? In response, nongovernmental action was taken first in 1919; this evolved into the Joint Commission on Accreditation of Hospitals in 1952.[16] Thus, information about hospitals is provided to potential users (or buyers of hospital service) through an emblem of approval, in spite of this indirect interference with free competition for the patient's patronage. Even so, an emblem of quality may not protect the consumer, since the hospital is ordinarily chosen not by him but by the doctor—who may (and often does) have his own reasons for selecting a nonaccredited facility.

Absence of Externalities

In the health sector, externalities abound with particular force. Each person's health status affects the health and welfare of everyone else. As a practical matter, therefore, nations at all stages of capitalist development have taken actions to assure the distribution of health care quite outside the mechanism of a free competitive market. One may not always appreciate the abandonment of laissez-faire dynamics that these actions constitute.

The rise of insurance for health care—first voluntary, later mandatory—was an early response to recognition of the societal importance of assured medical care at times of need. In the nineteenth century, as medical care became a market commodity (available only from charitable sources for the very poor and destitute), mutual insurance societies grew up in Europe to pay doctor bills for low-wage workers. Eventually in the 1880s, Germany enacted a law mandating "sickness insurance" for low-wage workers, and launching the concept of social security. Both the private and public forms of health care insurance spread to many other countries.[17] Not until 1965 did the United States enact any social insurance for general medical care, limiting it to the aged. Mandatory or social insurance constitutes a major adjustment to the problems of the free market ideology.[18] To a lesser extent, the same is true of voluntary health insurance. By spreading sickness risks over many people and over periods of time, the constraints of price on individual demand, when sickness strikes, are greatly reduced; the degree, of course, depends on the nature of co-payments, deductibles, and other "cost-sharing" requirements that may be imposed.[19] Prevention of insurance "abuse" by either patient or doctor—the so-called moral hazard of insurance—engenders all sorts of surveillance and policing in any insurance program. With all their weaknesses and faults, which are many, both voluntary health insurance and Medicare for the aged mollify the worst effects of the classical market mechanism in the distribution of medical care (albeit through introduction of another market for insurance).

To provide medical care for the poor—for those without even the low but stable incomes adequate for insurance—other adjustments have long been made. General revenue support of the U.S. Medicaid program is only the latest in a long saga of social measures to finance needed medical care that poor people were unable to purchase in the free market.[20] Parliamentary governments could ignore the brutalities of a market price for all care of the sick only at the risk of deaths in the street, mass rebellion, and social revolution. Compromising the free medical market, with tax-supported health care for the poor, was a much more prudent solution taken throughout the world, if only to maintain social order. The introduction of social security under Bismarck was not designed to extend democratic rights and liberties, but rather to weaken the rising socialist movement among European workers.[21]

The entire field of preventive medicine and public health has developed out of recognition of the crucial "externality" that each person's health care affects the well-being of all others. This has long been obvious for immunizations and other measures of communicable disease control; compulsory vaccinations, isolation, and quarantine have been implemented for centuries. Although less obvious, the same principle applies to health education on behavior to reduce the risk of chronic noncommunicable disease. We need not fall into the trap of blaming the victim for his "lifestyle" in recognizing the importance of social measures (e.g., bans on cigarette advertising) to discourage harmful habits.[22] Such social measures must operate not only outside the arena of free trade, but even as a frontal assault upon it.

These specific adjustments to the ill effects of a free market in the health sector may constitute enough empirical evidence of its grave inadequacies as a means for reasonable allocation of resources in society. All five of the conditions necessary for the market to serve as an efficient distributive mechanism are seriously lacking. But the ill effects of free trade and competition in the health sector are shown in other ways.

OTHER OUTCOMES OF FREE TRADE IN HEALTH CARE

The obstructive and antisocial rise of monopoly in the health sector has occurred again and again. Actions taken in response to this problem have led, in turn, to injurious secondary effects.

The U.S. pharmaceutical industry has engaged repeatedly in collusive price-fixing in restraint of trade. Convictions, such as that achieved for pegging the price of antibiotics to yield superprofits to several major firms after World War II, were widely publicized.[23] But such exposure of monopolistic practices is probably only the iceberg seen above the water. Is it not significant that the U.S. pharmaceutical industry has long had the highest rate of profit of any type of enterprise[24]—higher than the steel industry or the manufacture of computers?

Medical societies have long used "ethics" as a constraint against development of innovative patterns of medical care delivery. Their strategy has been essentially monopolistic. Agreements among producers to stifle innovation sabotaged the ability of competition to regulate the whole free enterprise system.

There were other more subtle ways, however, that private physicians could block the development of competitive new patterns of health care delivery, designed to give consumers a better deal. Consumer cooperatives getting their medical care through group practice clinics constituted one such pattern; doctors in these clinics could be barred from admitting their patients to community hospitals, dominated by private solo practitioners. Exactly such a tactic was used by the Medical Society of the District of Columbia, along with the American Medical Association, in an attempt to destroy the Group Health Association of Washington, D.C., in the 1930s. It took legal action in the courts to stop this assault on competition from new health care ideas, resulting in the 1943 conviction of the AMA for "criminal conspiracy in restraint of trade."[25] In spite of this watershed decision, medical societies continue to apply social ostracism and other subtle strategies against physicians who would deviate from the status quo of private fee-for-service medical practice.

The development of long-term contractual arrangements under free trade in the health sector has taken several forms. While constituting partial departures from conventional market arrangements, each of these mechanisms has generated secondary problems, which in turn require regulatory controls.

Recognition of broadly accessible health care as sound social policy led to the rise of health insurance—first voluntary and then mandatory—as discussed earlier. Insurance overcame the obstacles to accessibility erected by market prices for medical care; but, in the absence of regulation, it generated much unnecessary service to enhance the earnings of doctors and hospitals.

In reaction to this abuse—that is, a serious flaw in the very mechanism (health insurance) designed to adjust for the inequities caused by the free market—numerous corrective adjustments have become necessary. In most countries official fee schedules for medical services have been established, freezing price competition, and in the U.S. Medicare program various constraints have been put on the determination of "reasonable, customary, and prevailing" doctor fees. Under 1972 law, PSROs (professional standards review organizations) were set up throughout the nation to monitor the propriety of all services in hospitals financed by both Medicare and Medicaid.[26] It has also been found necessary to establish a federal Office of Fraud and Abuse, to cope with professional misconduct. Thus, socially planned insurance, organized to assure accessibility to health care, generates secondary problems, unless the economic freedom of vendors is regulated.

Health maintenance organizations (HMOs) are the most recent striking expression of a diversion to long-term contractual arrangements, in response to free market problems. The HMO is basically a strategy for complete removal from the orbit of the market of a population of patients and health care providers. Buyers and sellers make an agreement, a fixed-price contract, for future delivery (usually for one year) of needed medical care. This mechanism has been found to be so effective in controlling the cost escalations of the free medical market, that in 1973 federal legislation was enacted to promote it.[27] The growth of HMOs has been slower than some had hoped; the reasons are many, but a major one is doubtless the opposition of private medical entrepreneurs precisely because the HMO constitutes such a departure from free market dynamics. It greatly modifies the profit incentives to maximize sales. Moreover, the HMO is regarded as an incursion on physician freedom and a first step in a broader assault on the medical market.

At the same time, HMOs have not been an unmixed blessing; they have given rise to new forms of abuse. In the early 1970s, to reduce medical care expenditures for the poor, California and certain other states actively encouraged the establishment of HMOs for Medicaid-eligibles. But these "prepaid health plans" (PHPs) were allowed to operate without any official standards; as a result dozens of unscrupulous organizations were formed, giving seriously deficient services.[28] With fixed monthly payments from the state government assured, the PHPs gave grossly inadequate ambulatory as well as hospital care; an indigent patient would have to be at death's door before he was admitted to a hospital. It took widely publicized evidence of scandalous medical neglect or fiscal abuses to lead to new state regulation of these Medicaid HMOs. Only after this corrective action were the corrupt HMOs eliminated.[29]

Others have spoken glowingly of the HMO as the crucial strategy for achieving the benefits of free competition in the U.S. health care system.[30] The fundamental merit of the HMO concept is, in fact, its modification of the usual profit motive of maximizing the sale of medical services, toward an opposite motive of minimizing services—presumably through "maintenance of health." But the dynamic is far more complicated than this, and the potential for abuse is enormous, as shown in the California experience.

The allegedly effective competition among several HMOs in one Midwest metropolitan area has been widely acclaimed.[31] Its replication elsewhere or, indeed, its continued integrity in Minneapolis may be reasonably expected only if cautious state regulation and painstaking consumer education prevent the abuses experienced in California in the 1970s. (It is relevant that Minnesota's current statutory regulation of HMOs is especially rigorous.) Regulatory safeguards would be needed against still other potential abuses in "selection of risks" or "preferential pricing," which have long caused inequities in the commercial insurance industry.[32] Whether the burden of public regulation necessary to assure equity and efficiency—under a system of HMOs competing with each other and also with other health insurance programs—would be less than under a wholly planned health care system is very doubtful.

UNSOLVED PROBLEMS OF THE FREE MARKET

Beyond all the evidence of free market failure, reflected by the many adjustments stimulated in response, there are a host of persistent problems on which little action has been taken or the attempted corrections have been ineffective. Only some of the most prominent of these unsolved problems need be briefly noted.

High and endlessly rising costs of medical care are probably the most prominent unsolved problem in the whole contemporary health sector.[33] Several of the adjustments just reviewed have been directed to cost controls, but expenditures continue to mount. Some traditional economists argue that the regulatory constraints on competition are the *cause* of cost escalations—as though the many inherent obstacles to a free competitive market in health services, reviewed above, did not exist. The numerous imperfections of the competitive process in the health sector have not been sufficiently corrected by regulation, on the one hand, nor replaced by systematic planning, on the other. Prospective global budgeting of hospital operation, for example (not to be

confused with prospective *per diem* reimbursement), is not implement-
able in the current pluralistic American health economy. It is these
realities of halfway regulation, combined with halfway competition,
that yield inflation of health care costs.

While professional licensure has eliminated the worst chicanery
from the medical care market, it has not gone far enough. Disciplinary
actions taken against even grossly incompetent doctors are notoriously
weak. The beginnings of mandatory continuing education, enforced by
requirements for periodic relicensure of pharmacists, physicians,
nurses, and others in a few states, point up the need for great extension of
such policies.[34]

Excessive medical, and particularly surgical, specialization in
America has led to many difficulties, most prominently a serious shortage of primary care doctors. Under the Health Professions Educational
Assistance Act of 1976, training grants have been designed to favor
residencies in primary fields of medicine. Much more is needed, however, to assure the appropriate access of everyone to a continuing and
reliable source of primary health care.[35]

Geographic maldistribution of physicians and other health personnel—causing serious handicaps for rural populations—is a problem
plaguing the health care system of every capitalist nation. While many
factors account for this problem, the operation of the free market is
important among them; most rural people are relatively poor and lack the
purchasing power for proper medical care. Many countries have coped
with this by scrapping market mechanisms and requiring a period of
rural service from all new medical graduates. Norway has its highly
developed "district doctor" system, and the United States has its modest
"National Health Service Corps."[36] Far more powerful measures are
needed, if this major inequity of the free medical market is to be
corrected.

Permeating the American free market in health services is the
paradoxical problem of "supply creating demand"—fundamentally because the seller (doctor) rather than the buyer (patient) makes most of the
decisions on the health services to be obtained and paid for.[37] The
problem has been most conspicuous with respect to hospitalization and
its spiraling costs, and yet one wonders why it took until the late 1950s to
recognize the dynamics.

As the rise of U.S. hospital costs accelerated in the 1950s, attention
became focused on possible "overutilization." It was charged that,

because insurance had eliminated the constraints of price, patients were "abusing" it and consuming more hospital days than needed. One would have thought patients could check into a hospital, as into a hotel. Studies at Cornell's Institute of Hospital Administration, however, showed that—with almost any ratio of hospital beds in a community, high or low—doctors managed to keep those beds filled at about the same occupancy level.[38] As a result, New York State enacted in 1964 the first "certificate of need" law to control hospital bed supply. Soon many other states did the same, and federal law in 1974 made such regulation virtually nationwide.[8] What a strange commentary on the operations of the free market model of supply, demand, competition, and price! Excess supply did not bring down the price, but caused greater overall expenditures.

Indeed, excess hospital beds have resulted not only in higher rates of patient-day utilization, but even higher costs per day, as competing hospitals acquire superfluous technology in order to attract doctors. How can more CT (computerized tomography) scanners be justified in Los Angeles County (some 65 units for a population of 7,000,000) than in all of Great Britain (population of 55,000,000) where the machine was invented?[39] The low point in hospital enticements to doctors may have been reached in May 1980, when evidence was disclosed that a supposedly prestigious institution, with low bed occupancy, was operating a "call girl service" for doctors, to induce them to admit patients.[40] Legal prosecution, of course, was necessary. With respect to CT scanners or excess hospital beds, planning agency decisions—hardly distinguishable from regulation—are necessary to control the extravagances of the free market in hospital care. Not many states, however, have been as forthright as Michigan in passing legislation to deliberately reduce excess hospital capacity.[41]

Evidence that supply creates demand has now accumulated for every component of the health care industry, not only for the use of hospital beds.[42] Surgeons create "demand" for surgical operations, the benefits of which are far from established.[43] In Canada, the in-migration of foreign medical graduates was stopped a few years ago when it was learned that each new physician meant an expenditure of some $300,000—about 40 percent for his own gross income and 60 percent for the hospital and other secondary services that he generated. Similarly, a steady increase in the U.S. doctor–population ratio has led not to any decline in prices, but to a rise in aggregate expenditures.

Partial or halfway planning leaves many problems unsolved. Thus collectivized financing along with entrepreneurial delivery of service creates enormous problems in surveillance of quality and expenditures. For reasons explored earlier, insurance, taxation, and other third-party sources of finance have been mobilized everywhere to help achieve health care equity. At the same time, everyone agrees that third-party payment inevitably dulls or eliminates both the doctor's and the patient's sensitivity to price. Such social financing, nevertheless, is quite properly designed to facilitate the seeking of health service in the first place. Thus, for the lion's share of total health care costs now supported by third parties, the free market has already been largely abandoned.[44] Yet monitoring medical care fee claims under third-party financing programs is enormously difficult and seldom effective.

Within the field of health insurance, insofar as competition operates among carriers, its effects have promoted inequity. The commercial insurance practice of "experience-rating"—decreasing premiums for the young and healthy, and increasing them for the aged and disabled—has forced the nonprofit insurance plans to follow suit or lose their enrollment.[45] The only solution to this perverse dynamics would be a system of universal social financing, within a framework of either enormously regulated competition or systematic social planning.

Zealous devotion to concepts of the free market and competition has led to the rejection of "ethical" bans on medical advertising.[46] The importance of consumer accessibility to complete objective information is one thing; freedom of advertising is another. Even with the utmost scientific effort, evaluation of either the "process" or "outcome" of health services is extremely difficult to carry out, let alone to report lucidly. Take note of the limited impact of the U.S. Federal Trade Commission on the advertising of so-called ethical drugs—as revealed each month in the highly authoritative *Medical Letter on Drugs and Therapeutics*—in spite of the relatively broad powers vested in government by the Food, Drug, and Cosmetic Act. Objective information should be broadcast by government or some neutral body, not by parties obviously trying to sell their own particular products. Are we to welcome to the health care industry the skillful distortions with which advertising has glamorized cigarette smoking, liquor consumption, and other garden paths to disease and death?

Inadequate consumer information persists in plaguing a free market health care model, despite the most earnest efforts to ameliorate it through education. To the extent that a patient may have an impact on the doctor's decisions, he must be inordinately knowledgeable. Even if he or she is, it is rare for the patient to prevail over the judgment of the doctor. Not many patients are as sophisticated as Norman Cousins who, aided by a physician of exceptional humility, cured himself of an incurable disease.[47] For every Mr. Cousins, there are thousands of other patients whose noncompliance with their doctor's prescription of antihypertensive drugs, for example, leads to fatal strokes.

The problems arising from the complexity of medical information, beyond the understanding of the vast majority of consumers, can be tragic. The choice of a faulty product (e.g., an incompetent doctor) may be prolonged disability or death. Rapid technological change creates new information requirements almost daily. If new drugs could freely enter the market each week, there could be endless human tragedy and waste as consumers tested each product. (Regulation, of course, has been necessary to bar this.) Even after a product has been purchased and consumed, how can the consumer judge its value? Health outcomes depend on many environmental, genetic, and other factors outside of medical care.

Market mechanisms may achieve reasonable distribution of some luxury goods and services, such as fancy clothing or nightclub entertainment, but they cannot be expected to work soundly for health care. Regarding services accounting for 80–90 percent of health care costs, decisions in the last analysis are made by the doctor, not the patient. How can one expect *consumer* preferences to govern the flow of products in the medical market?[48]

Finally, one need only take note of the magnitude of "unfinished business" formerly faced by the nation's 212 local health planning agencies to recognize the enormity of health deficiencies remaining in the free market of health care. It has not been excessive regulation, but the consequences of the free market that led to establishment of Health Systems Agencies as mechanisms to cope with excess general hospital beds, health care cost-containment, emergency medical services, environmental health protection, perinatal intensive care, and rehabilitation services—to name only some of the problems recently identified in the planning of one local HSA.[49]

Health planning (national and local) constitutes, after all, a series of interventions in the free market of health care, designed to correct its many failures.

COMMERCIALIZATION OF HEALTH SERVICES

In the last decade or so the impact of free trade and competition on the U.S. health care system has had especially alarming effects. For years a small fraction of American hospitals have been operated for profit—that is, they are the 14 percent of short-term general hospitals that in 1976 contained 8 percent of the beds. With escalating costs, however, many hospitals of all sponsorships ran into difficulties in the 1970s and 1980s; one response was the organization of corporations for the ownership and operation of numerous hospitals, in order to acquire economies of scale and managerial efficiency.[50]

These corporate chains of hospitals have begun to grow rapidly. By 1982, proprietary hospitals—after declining in number for many years—increased to 773, or about 15 percent of all general hospitals, with 10.4 percent of the general hospital beds. About half of all these facilities (now often called "investor-owned hospitals") are owned by large corporations operating chains of institutions. In addition, the hospital chain corporations have contracts for the management of about 300 voluntary nonprofit hospitals, and even some public hospitals. Most of the facilities are small or medium-sized and are located in the sunbelt states and in suburban communities, where economic conditions are relatively prosperous.

In spite of frequent claims, studies have shown no evidence of greater efficiency in the operation of these for-profit hospitals. They have evidently been successful in collecting payments from both private insurance and government payers, and their charges are substantially higher—particularly for ancillary services. A careful California study showed that total charges for service in the for-profit hospitals were 24 percent higher than in comparable voluntary hospitals, and collections were 10 percent higher. As businesses, the corporate chains have been so profitable that several of them have sold stock on the New York Stock Exchange, enabling them to amass capital for further expansion.[51]

Other sections of the health care field have shown similar signs of commercialization. Nursing homes for long-term care have long been predominantly under proprietary ownership (about 77 percent of 19,000 facilities), but now an enlarging fraction have come under the control of large corporations. Agencies operating home care programs have traditionally been offshoots of nonprofit hospitals or charitable associations for visiting nurse service, but all this is changing. About 10 large corporations have bought up or established hundreds of these agencies and have come to control an expanding share of the field. Clinical laboratories are still another health resource, numbering in the thousands, and about one-third of these have been acquired by for-profit corporations. Most are independent laboratories, using the mails or messenger services, but some are even in hospitals.[52]

Still other health services have become the basis of for-profit businesses. There are mobile CT (computerized tomography) scanners, cardiopulmonary testing machines, dental care programs, weight-control clinics, and alcohol treatment programs. Hemodialysis for end-stage renal disease (a service financed by Medicare) has been especially attractive to private investors, and in 1980 about 40 percent of this service was provided by a handful of large for-profit corporations. Staffing and operating emergency rooms in hospitals has even been taken up as a corporate activity, with several large companies selling complete "E.R. packages" to hundreds of hospitals.

Why, one may ask, should this increasing commercialization of the U.S. health care system be a matter of concern? Entrepreneurial advocates argue that selling stock is a sound way of raising money for capital expansion, and large-size operations yield economies of scale and other efficiencies. Moreover, the profit motive has long fueled the pharmaceutical industry, and for that matter, the ordinary private practitioner of medicine or dentistry is engaged in a small for-profit enterprise. But there are differences.

The drug industry, by reason of its entire entrepreneurial history, has generated a large body of regulation at the federal and state levels. Much human tragedy lies in back of that legislation, which has ameliorated the industry's worst abuses. Medical and dental practice is to some degree controlled by ethical codes which have evolved over the centuries. In hospitals, medical staff bylaws impose many constraints on the physician's behavior, and numerous government or insurance programs review the work for which a doctor seeks payment. Even so, the private practice of medicine is replete with problems, ranging from extravagant and unnecessary procedures to faulty performance sufficiently serious to warrant thousands of malpractice suits.

Commercialization of hospitals, nursing homes, home care programs, clinical laboratories, and so on introduces the profit motive on a much larger scale. Each of these involves a complex series of activities, in which the potential abuses, to aggrandize earnings, are tremendous. The array of services that might be rendered to a hospital or nursing home patient, each for a price, is almost endless. The incentives to a home care program or any facility serving patients is to accept the "easy" case, on which profits can be high, and reject the case—simple or complex—on which payment is questionable. If dividends are to be paid to stockholders, what incentive is there for a hospital to operate an outpatient clinic for the poor, to conduct continuing education for doctors, or to carry out clinical research? Such nonremunerative activities are, indeed, very rare in for-profit hospitals.

The entire role of the health services as a social function for the improvement of human welfare is frontally challenged by the profit motive. Except perhaps for drug production, every component of health care systems in the United States and in the entire world has been undergoing social change toward becoming an organized public service. More and more doctors, in America and elsewhere, have become employed in government programs or within other organized frameworks. Hospitals in most countries are predominantly public, and becoming more so. The scope of public health is expanding, and organized health services for children, for industrial workers, for aged and disabled persons, for the mentally ill are winning the increasing attention of governments at all points in the political spectrum. Professional education is increasingly supported by public authorities, and medical research is financed overwhelmingly by tax funds. The financing of health care, preventive and curative, is predominantly a collectivized or social process in all developed countries, including the United States.

In this national and international environment, the current wave of commercialization in the United States can only be regarded as anomalous and probably temporary. The regulations that are bound to be generated to protect quality and to contain costs will have to be increasingly probing and burdensome. If only in the interests of economy and the reduction of regulatory bureaucracy, the historic trend of health service, evolving from a market commodity toward a social right, is almost certain to continue in the long run.

CONCLUSION—SYSTEMATIC SOCIAL PLANNING OF THE HEALTH SECTOR

We trust this is enough of a recitation of the failures, distortions, wastages, and human inequities of the free market in health care to clarify our reasons for rejecting it, and preferring a strategy of *systematic social planning*. The failures of a free market in health care to achieve effective allocation of resources for meeting the needs of populations have been gigantic. Some entrepreneurial voices even reject as "naive" the very concept of *needs,* and wish only to consider "effective demand" in a market. Yet the market has not been completely abandoned in capitalist nations, only because countless corrective measures have kept patching it up.

Entitlement to health care, unlike most other goods and services, has come to be recognized throughout the world as a "universal human right."[53] The rationale is both humane and pragmatic. To implement its distribution, one cannot be satisfied with a free market mechanism that treats health care fundamentally as a commodity to be produced for profit and sold. A pig trough philosophy of access has been rejected. The incompatibilities between these two concepts of health care—as a commodity for sale versus a basic right—are overwhelming.

In broad terms, an agenda for a systematically planned health care system is not difficult to summarize: (1) universal population coverage; (2) comprehensive services, based solely on need; (3) emphasis on prevention through integration with treatment; (4) health personnel trained at public expense to serve in coordinated teams; (5) health facilities public and regionalized; (6) quality regulated through built-in organizational structure (rather than external surveillance); and (7) fully collectivized financing.[54] In a word, a planned social system would replace the vagaries of the competitive medical market. Consumer choice would not disappear (e.g., for Doctor A rather than Doctor B), but it would be constrained by conditions under which one person's choice does not thwart reasonable response to another person's need.

The way of science, which matured only after the days of Adam Smith, has far more effective strategies to offer, both along the biological and the social dimensions of health care. Health services can be effectively distributed, not by the tools of price or non-price competition, not on the basis of personal affluence, geographical location, social position, educational sophistication, or any other of the features on which free market dynamics depend. The production and distribution of health services can be based on their scientifically demonstrated value and on the differential needs of each human being.[55]

The strategies required to construct a soundly planned health care system are not simple, nor free from the possibilities of error. Each of the above seven attributes of such a system requires vast information and sophisticated judgment in the arena of both economics and politics. If one prefers an option of modifying the free market, however, the requirements for regulatory intervention are no less—if efficiency and social justice are to be attained. Programs of this sort, formulated by Alain Enthoven[30] and others, would require elaborate administration and constant regulation. These complex issues and options must be discussed, but the issue before us is the past and present medical markets. We believe it can be demonstrated that deliberate and systematic social planning of the health services can be more effective, less subject to the evils of corruption and inequity, than the most judiciously regulated model of the free competitive market. The lessons of history on the perverse social consequences of the pursuit of individual self-interest in the health sector are abundant. The human and social benefits of rational scientific health planning are demonstrable throughout the modern world.

In this chapter, we have addressed the ascending wave of opinion in the United States that current difficulties in the health sector arise from "too much" regulation, and that the path to efficiency and justice lies in uninhibited competition and free trade. An objective assessment of past experience, we believe, points to a path in exactly the opposite direction.

REFERENCES

1. Levin A (Ed.): Regulating Health Care: The Struggle for Control. New York: Academy of Political Science, 1980.
2. See, for example, Mansfield E: Economics (3rd ed.). New York: Norton, 1980. Also Varian H: Microeconomic Analysis. New York: Norton, 1978.
3. Center for Community Health Systems: Community Hospitals and the Challenge of Primary Care. New York: Columbia University, 1975.
4. Roemer MI: Primary care and physician extenders in affluent countries. Int J Health Serv 1977; 7(4):545–555.
5. McCarthy EG, Widmer GW: Effects of screening by consultants on recommended elective surgical procedures. N Engl J Med 1974; 291:1331–1335.
6. Kessler MS: Physician compensation: Survey shows marked increase in contractual arrangements. The Hospital Medical Staff, July 1976; 19–25.
7. Bridgman RF, Roemer MI: Hospital Legislation and Hospital Systems. WHO Public Health Paper No. 50, Geneva, 1973.
8. Rosenfeld LS, Rosenfeld I: National health planning in the United States: Prospects and portents. Int J Health Serv 1975; 5(3):441–453.

9. Roemer R, Roemer MI: Health Manpower Policies in the Belgian Health Care System. Washington, DC: U.S. Health Resources Administration, DHEW Pub. (HRA) 77–38, 1977.

10. Goodman LJ, Bennett TH, Oden RJ: Group Medical Practice in the United States, 1975. Chicago: American Medical Association, 1976.

11. Roemer R: Legal systems regulating health personnel: A comparative analysis. Milbank Mem Fund Q 1968; 56:431.

12. Wardwell WJ: The future of chiropractic. N Engl J Med 1980; 302:688–690.

13. U.S. Health Resources Administration: State Regulation of Health Manpower. Washington, DC: 1977. DHEW Pub. No. (HRA) 77–49.

14. Stern BJ: Social Factors and Medical Progress. Princeton: Princeton University Press, 1941.

15. Anderson O, Young J, Jansen W: The government and the consumer: Evolution of food and drug laws. J Public Law 1964; 13:189.

16. Roemer MI, Friedman JW: Doctors in Hospitals: Medical Staff Organization and Hospital Performance. Baltimore: Johns Hopkins Press, 1971.

17. Roemer MI: Organization of Medical Care under Social Security. Geneva: International Labour Office, 1969.

18. Feingold E: Medicare: Policies and Politics. San Francisco: Chandler, 1966.

19. Maynard A: Pricing, demanders, and the supply of health care. Int J Health Serv 1979; 9(1):121–133.

20. Stern BJ: Medical Services by Government: Local, State, and Federal. New York: Commonwealth Fund, 1946.

21. Sigerist HE: From Bismarck to Beveridge: Developments and trends in social security legislation. Bull Hist Med April 1943; 8:365–388.

22. Crawford R: You are dangerous to your health: The ideology and politics of victim blaming. Int J Health Serv 1977; 7(4):663–679.

23. Silverman MM, Lee PR: Pills, Profits, and Politics. Berkeley: University of California Press, 1974.

24. Harris SE: The Economics of American Medicine. New York: Macmillan, 1964.

25. Hansen HE: Group health plans—A twenty year legal review. Minnesota Law Review, March 1958.

26. Gosfield A: PSROs: The Law and the Health Consumer. Cambridge, Mass.: Ballinger, 1975.

27. Federal Trade Commission: The Health Maintenance Organization and Its Effects on Competition. Washington, DC, 1977. Also McClure W: On broadening the definition of and removing regulatory barriers to a competitive health care system. J Health Politics, Policy Law Fall 1978; 3:303–327.

28. D'Onofrio CN, Mullen PD: Consumer problems with prepaid health plans in California. Public Health Rep. April 1977; 92:121–134.

29. Roemer MI: Better weather ahead for California's prepaid health plans. Impact: American Medical News 1976; 19(42):7–8.

30. Enthoven AC: Consumer choice health plan (in two parts). N Engl J Med 23 and 30 March, 1978; 298:650–658, 709–720.

31. Christianson JB, McClure W: Competition in the delivery of medical care. N Engl J Med 11 October 1979; 301:812–818.

32. American Public Health Association: Health maintenance organizations: A policy paper. Am J Public Health December 1971; 61:2528–2536.

33. Schweitzer SO (Ed): Policies for the Containment of Health Care Costs and Expenditures. Washington, DC: US Public Health Service, Fogarty International Center, 1978.

34. Derbyshire RC: In: Hearings on Health Professions Educational Assistance Act of 1974. Washington, DC: US Senate Committee on Labor and Public Welfare, 93rd Congress, 2nd Session, 1974.

35. Richmond J: Currents in American Medicine. Cambridge, Mass.: Harvard University Press, 1969.

36. Roemer MI: Strategies for increasing rural medical manpower in five industrialized countries. Public Health Rep March–April 1978; 93:142–146.

37. Roemer MI: Editorial: Hospital utilization and the health care system. Am J Public Health October 1976; 66:953–955.

38. Roemer MI, Shain M: Hospital Utilization under Insurance. Chicago: American Hospital Association (Hospital Monograph Series No. 6), 1959.

39. State of California Department of Health: Computed Tomographic Scanners in California as of September 8, 1977. Sacramento, 1978.

40. Lonsdale J, Malnic E: Medical officials arrested in sex case. Los Angeles Times, 30 May 1980.

41. Comprehensive Health Planning Council of Southeastern Michigan: Annual Implementation Plan 1980. Detroit, 1980.

42. Evans RG: Supplier-induced demand: Some empirical evidence and implications. In Perlman M (Ed): The Economics of Health and Medical Care, London: Macmillan, 1974; 162–173.

43. Lewis CE: Variations in the incidence of surgery. N Engl J Med 16 October 1969; 880–884.

44. Newhouse JP: The structure of health insurance and the erosion of competition in the marketplace. In Greenberg W (Ed): Competition in the Health Care Sector. Washington, DC: Federal Trade Commission, 1978; 270–278.

45. McIntyre D: Voluntary Health Insurance and Ratemaking. Ithaca, N.Y.: Cornell University Press, 1962.

46. Sloan FA: Competition among physicians. In Greenberg W (Ed): Competition in the Health Care Sector. Washington, DC: Federal Trade Commission, 1978; 57–131.

47. Cousins N: Anatomy of an illness (as perceived by the patient). N Engl J Med 23 December 1976; 295:1458–1463.

48. Kelman S: Laying on the invisible hand: Ideology in health economics. Int J Health Serv 1980; 10(4):703–709.

49. Comprehensive Health Planning Council of Southeastern Michigan: Health Systems Plan for Southeastern Michigan 1980 through 1984. Detroit, October 1979.

50. Relman AS: The new medical-industrial complex. N Engl J Med 23 October 1980; 303:963–970.

51. Pattison RV, Katz HM: Investor-owned and not-for-profit hospitals. N Engl J Med 11 August 1983; 309:347–353.

52. Ermann D, Gabel J: Multihospital systems: Issues and empirical findings. Health Affairs Spring 1984; 3:50–64.
53. World Health Organization: The Declaration of Alma Ata. Geneva, 1979.
54. Roemer MI: An ideal health care system for America. In Strauss Al (Ed): Where Medicine Falls. New Brunswick, NJ: Trans-Action Books, 1973; 77–93.
55. Institute of Medicine: Health Planning in the United States: Issues in Guideline Development. Washington, DC: National Academy of Sciences, 1980.

Chapter **7**

Committee on the Costs of Medical Care and the Drive for National Health Insurance

On October 4, 1984 the American movement for national health insurance lost its most profound analyst and most eloquent advocate, when the life of I. S. Falk came to an end. In the more than half-century of work of I. S. Falk, one finds a remarkably accurate reflection of the social battles to achieve a program of economic support to make essential health services available to the entire U.S. population. Some have spoken of these battles as a "lost reform,"[1] but the movement is still alive, and a review of Falk's life and the events around it suggest far more gains than losses. The American health care movement, to which Falk contributed so much, has been a story of unquestionable progress, in spite of the distance still to be covered to reach its ultimate goal.

I.S. FALK: ADVOCATE OF NATIONAL HEALTH INSURANCE

Isadore S. Falk was born in Brooklyn, New York, in 1899.[2] In 1915, he became a laboratory assistant to C.-E. A. Winslow, the newly appointed Professor of Public Health at Yale Medical School. From this time on,

Falk's life falls into five periods, only the highlights of which can be given here.

The first period, 1915–1929, was essentially biological; in 1923 Falk earned the Ph.D. at Yale in public health, working in bacteriology and immunology. From 1923 to 1929, he taught hygiene and bacteriology at the University of Chicago, advancing from Assistant Professor to full Professor.

The second period, 1929–1935, comprised Falk's highly productive years with the Committee on the Costs of Medical Care, with some follow-up work. The Committee had been formed with foundation support in 1927, and when Falk received an invitation to join it, the entire character of his life was changed. Soon he was appointed Associate Director of the research staff and became immersed in the socioeconomic aspects of sickness and medical care in America. (Throughout the rest of his life many people thought that Falk's basic discipline was economics.)

In the third period, 1936–1953, Dr. Falk served in the federal government, first as Assistant Director, then in 1940 as Director of the Bureau of Research and Statistics of the Social Security Board (later Social Security Administration). From this position, he was appointed to several federal committees that played major roles in the formulation of U.S. federal policy and strategy on national health insurance and related issues. The first of these was the Technical Committee on Medical Care of the Interdepartmental Committee on Health and Welfare Activities, appointed by President Franklin D. Roosevelt in 1937. The Technical Committee drew up in 1938 the specifications for "A National Health Program," which became the framework for legislative proposals later introduced in the U.S. Congress by Senator Robert F. Wagner.

The "National Health Program" called for five measures: (1) grants to the states for mandatory health insurance, (2) grants to the states for medical care to welfare recipients plus the medically indigent, (3) federal permanent disability insurance, (4) grants-in-aid for hospital construction, and (5) grants to the states for expanding public health and particularly child health programs. The Wagner National Health Bill embodying these proposals was brought before Congress in early 1939, on the eve of World War II in Europe. (Although the War thwarted any legislative action at this time, within the next two decades, all but the first of these five proposals became enacted into law.)

After the War, in 1945, similar multipurpose legislation—drafted in large part by Falk and his staff—was again introduced in Congress. The first Presidential message to Congress on health and health insurance (by Harry Truman in November 1945) was drafted largely by Falk, as were subsequent versions of national health insurance acts (the Wagner-Murray-Dingell Bills) in 1947 and 1949.

With the election in 1952 of a conservative federal administration, under President Dwight Eisenhower, the idea of comprehensive national health insurance seemed hopeless, and Falk drafted a proposal for health insurance limited to aged beneficiaries of Social Security. A few years later this was introduced in Congress by Representative Aimes Forand, and it went through several versions before its enactment as "medical care for the aged" or Medicare in 1965. In December 1953, with the new federal atmosphere unfriendly to social legislation, Falk resigned from the government.

During the fourth period in I. S. Falk's life, 1954–1961, he served as an independent consultant on health services planning and organization. This was initially on studies for international agencies (in Malaya and Singapore, Panama and the Canal Zone), but later, mainly for the United Steel Workers of America as their analyst and consultant on union health care programs.

The fifth period, 1961–1979, saw Dr. Falk back in New Haven, where his life as a health professional had started. From 1961 to 1968, he served as professor of public health (medical care) in the reorganized Yale Department of Epidemiology and Public Health. On retirement from Yale, he immediately undertook the organization of the Community Health Care Center Plan, which began operation in 1971. Falk was its Executive Director, and the plan became the first fully qualified health maintenance organization in the nation, under the 1973 federal HMO Act. When he retired in 1979, Falk had built a program of organized medical care combined with health insurance, which embodied several of the principles advocated by the Committee on the Costs of Medical Care almost 50 years earlier.

Throughout the 1970s, Falk served on the Committee for National Health Insurance, organized by the President of the United Auto Workers, Walter Reuther. As head of the Technical Committee of this body, he returned again to the turbulent waters of national health insurance. It was this committee that did the basic drafting of the Health Security Act, introduced by Senator Edward Kennedy in 1971. The Kennedy Bill generated during the 1970s introduction of some 23 other health insurance bills, representing a very broad range of political views.[3] There was widespread talk that the nation faced a "health care crisis" and that "national health insurance was an idea whose time had come." Yet, with the election of Ronald Reagan in 1980, NHI again became a dead issue, and Dr. Falk did not live to see achievement of the goal for which he had fought so long and hard.

FRUSTRATION OR PROGRESS?

In spite of the frustrations in the struggle for national health insurance, reflected in the life of I. S. Falk, I suggested at the outset that the American health care movement has been a story of unquestionable progress. Is this interpretation valid? Several historians have challenged the widespread concept of "progress" in any large social development, and have claimed that this view of major trends distorts reality according to the wishes of the observer. They have labeled this view as the fallacy of "historicism," which has been criticized for many years;[4] it has recently been defined as "the belief that there is a purpose in history which it is our professional duty to discover and communicate."[5]

Interpretation of the half-century from 1929 to 1979—the salient years of I. S. Falk's life—is an appropriate test of historicism. Were the events of these years *mainly* a saga of frustration or of progress? As in the basic sciences, the crucial task is to ask the right question. It has been wisely said in biology that if one asks Nature the right question, one never gets the wrong answer. In the issue before us, should we ask: "Why has the United States failed to enact statutory national health insurance?" Or should we ask: "What has happened with respect to the provision of health services to the American people?"

If we pose the second question in a time frame of about the last 50 years—let us say from 1930 to 1980—the answer can be given with an abundance of factual data, and with little need for conjecture. This question is, of course, a large one, and needs to be subdivided to be answered. An extremely useful method of subdivision is to examine the specific recommendations of the Committee on the Costs of Medical Care (CCMC), to which I. S. Falk made so large a contribution. The last of the 27 volumes produced by the CCMC is entitled *Medical Care for the American People* and contains the Committee's final recommendations. These clearly emerge from the findings of the extensive studies on the health of the U.S. population, its receipt of health services, its expenditures (costs), and related matters. The recommendations are designed to solve or reduce the problems identified.

THE CCMC AND ITS RECOMMENDATIONS

The Committee on the Costs of Medical Care was organized in 1927 "to study the economic aspects of the care and prevention of illness" in the United States.[6] The members represented private medical practice, public health, diverse institutions, special groups from the social sciences, and the general population. The Committee was chaired by Dr. Ray Lyman Wilbur, a former president of the American Medical Association and at the time Secretary of the Interior under President Herbert Hoover. Its initial Study Director was Harry H. Moore, to whom I. S. Falk was Associate Director in charge of research for the last three years, 1929–1932, of the Committee's five-year existence.

With so broad a composition, it is no surprise that the Committee did not reach unanimity in its final recommendations, and that two minority reports—from private physicians and dentists on the Committee—were issued. The majority report contained five major recommendations, and numerous subsidiary proposals offering detailed suggestions on how each recommendation might be implemented. The major recommendations were so prescient that they should be quoted in full. Each began with "The Committee recommends that . . ." and continued as follows:[7]

1. Medical service, both preventive and therapeutic, should be furnished largely by organized groups of physicians, dentists, nurses, pharmacists, and other associated personnel. Such groups should be organized, preferably around a hospital, for rendering complete home, office, and hospital care. The form of organization should encourage the maintenance of high standards and the development or preservation of a personal relation between patient and physician.
2. All basic public health services—whether provided by governmental or nongovernmental agencies—[should be extended] so that they will

be available to the entire population according to its needs. Primarily this extension requires increased financial support for official health departments and full-time trained health officers and members of their staffs whose tenure is dependent only upon professional and administrative competence.

3. The costs of medical care [should] be placed on a group payment basis, through the use of insurance, through the use of taxation, or through the use of both these methods. This is not meant to preclude the continuation of medical service on an individual fee basis for those who prefer the present method. Cash benefits, i.e., compensation for wage-loss due to illness, if and when provided, should be separate and distinct from medical services.

4. The study, evaluation, and coordination of medical service [should] be considered important functions for every state and local community, that agencies [should] be formed to exercise these functions, and that the coordination of rural with urban services [should] receive special attention.

5. In the field of professional education: (A) the training of physicians [should] give increasing emphasis to the teaching of health and the prevention of disease; more effective efforts [should] be made to provide trained health officers; the social aspects of medical practice [should] be given greater attention; specialties [should] be restricted to those specially qualified; and postgraduate educational opportunities [should] be increased; (B) dental students [should] be given a broader educational background; (C) pharmaceutical education [should] place more stress on the pharmacist's responsibilities and opportunities for public service; (D) nursing education [should] be thoroughly remoulded to provide well-educated and well-qualified registered nurses; (E) less thoroughly trained but competent nursing aides or attendants [should] be provided; (F) adequate training for nurse-midwives [should] be provided; and (G) opportunities [should] be offered for the systematic training of hospital and clinic administrators.

It soon became obvious that recommendations 1 and 3 were the most contentious, although in retrospect one may be struck with the great cautiousness of their wording. The clause in recommendation 3, that it was "not meant to preclude the continuation of medical service on an individual fee basis for those who prefer the present method," meant advocacy of *voluntary* insurance, but this did not spare the Committee report from vitriolic attacks by the American Medical Association.

To cast light on the central question about the developments for provision of medical care to the American people over the last 50 years, since the CCMC report, it will be helpful to consider separately each of the five recommendations. What has actually happened?

ORGANIZATION OF MEDICAL SERVICES

At the time of the CCMC report, the nearly universal pattern for providing medical services in America was through the private offices of individual medical practitioners. The deficiencies of such isolated medical work, in relation to the increasing complexity of medical science and technology, were expounded by the Committee as the basis for its first recommendation. Applying the definition of "group practice" used by the American Medical Association (three or more physicians working together, with ancillary personnel, and sharing income in some prearranged manner), in 1932 only 0.9 percent of active non-federal physicians in the United States were in group practice.[8] By 1975, this proportion had grown to 18.5 percent. Using a denominator of non-federal *office-based* physicians, in 1980 the proportion in group practice was 46 percent.[9]

Independent group medical practice was not the form of organization most highly favored by the Committee. It advocated that medical groups "should be organized, preferably around a hospital. . . ." But, as we will find for the other recommendations, in assessment of a 50-year trend, the form in which an idea is implemented can hardly be expected to correspond precisely to an initial idea. The gradual replacement of solo practice by group practice is clearly observable in American ambulatory medical care, and this is surely evidence of progress in the organization of medical services. This judgment remains valid, even though about half the medical groups, with about one-third of the group doctors, are single-specialty rather than multispecialty in makeup.

In enlarging on its first recommendation, the CCMC speaks of the organization of "community medical centers" (through hospitals or as satellites to hospitals), industrial medical services, university medical programs, private group clinics (equivalent to "group practices"), physicians' private offices in hospitals, and other modalities. The Committee also advocates the greater use of "subsidiary personnel," including nurse-midwives, of organized nursing service (as against private-duty nursing), "pay clinics" attached to hospitals, and so on.

With the possible exception of midwifery, in which advancement has been relatively small, progress is observable in all these sectors. Students in the vast majority of colleges and universities are now served by organized health care programs.[10] Occupational health services in industry have developed only moderately in small plants (100 workers or less), but in larger plants—where the majority of workers are now employed—the trend has clearly been toward increasingly comprehensive organized services.[11] The organization of "pay clinics" in hospitals for non-indigent patients has not taken the form envisaged by the Committee, but the enormous expansion of hospital outpatient services, for both paying and publicly subsidized patients, is surely a movement in the same direction. The rates of utilization of hospital outpatient departments for emergency care, for referred private patients, and for scheduled clinics have been steadily upward. Regarding the strong orientation of the first CCMC recommendation toward hospitals, it may also be noted that the general medical staff organization of these facilities has become more and more rigorous, and the full-time employment of doctors by hospitals has become increasingly common.[12]

STRENGTHENING OF PUBLIC HEALTH SERVICES

The thrust of the CCMC's second recommendation is for the extension of organized preventive health services, which are specified as vital statistics, environmental sanitation, communicable disease control, laboratory services, maternal and child hygiene, health education, dental care for children, and the control of tuberculosis, venereal disease, hookworm infestation, and other endemic diseases. The Committee takes pains to say that these services may be "provided by governmental or non-governmental agencies."

The progress in this field since 1930 has been beyond question. With the rise and expansion of federal grants-in-aid to the states for public health and related services after 1935, the size and scope of state and local public health agencies increased greatly. The growth of responsibilities of the federal U.S. Public Health Service has been even greater.[13] This expansion of public programs applied not only to the traditional preventive services specified by the CCMC, but also to the medical care of crippled children, the planning and subsidy of hospital construction, the establishment of mental health clinics, the community control of heart disease, cancer, and other chronic disorders, the licensure of hospitals and nursing homes, and the provision of general primary health care. At the national level, Public Health Service responsibilities have come to include the subsidy of health professional education and the performance as well as financial support of biomedical research on all major disease problems.

After 1965, it is true that most of the continued expansion of public responsibilities for health, for both prevention and therapy, was implemented through agencies other than the "official health departments." For many political reasons, community ("neighborhood") health centers and other health programs for the poor were developed through grants from the independent U.S. Office of Economic Opportunity to various local citizen groups. When Medicare and Medicaid (see below) were enacted in 1965, their administration was turned over mainly to private insurance carriers and to state departments of welfare. The Regional Medical Program for Heart Disease, Cancer and Stroke (RMP) and the Comprehensive Health Planning (CHP) program were administered nationally by the U.S. Public Health Service, but locally RMP functioned mainly through medical schools and CHP through new and mainly nongovernmental agencies.

Nevertheless, the 50-year trend has been toward increased *social* responsibility for health services, both preventive and therapeutic. Even though official health departments have been supplemented by several other public and private entities, responsibility for more and more aspects of health promotion and medical care has been transferred from the individual to organized groups. Indeed, since about 1970, the health department's classical central mission of disease prevention and health promotion has come to permeate the entire health care system of the United States. Public health agencies have come to see as their major role, not to provide selected preventive health services directly, but to stimulate and educate all participants in the health care system to stress prevention and healthful "lifestyles" in their daily work.[14]

GROUP PAYMENT FOR MEDICAL SERVICES

To many, the third recommendation of the CCMC was the most radical and controversial of all, because it was widely believed that organized group financing of medical care would lead eventually to many crucial changes in the way medicine was practiced. Individual practitioners, hospitals, pharmacists, and other health care providers all feared that "he who pays the piper calls the tune," and they expected that any organized group that paid for health services would soon be telling doctors and others how to practice their professions. The potential reduction of incomes was some cause for apprehension, but even greater was the fear of an assault on professional independence.

In calling for group payment for health service, through insurance, taxation, or both, the CCMC took pains to refer to numerous specific programs that had already voluntarily applied such mechanisms. It spoke of voluntary cooperative health insurance, required health insurance for low-income groups, aid by local governments for health insurance, salaried or subsidized physicians in rural areas, state and federal aid, voluntary hospital insurance, tax funds for local hospital service, tax funds for medical care of indigent, and public support for the cure of chronic diseases. "None of these recommendations," the Committee said, "involves an untried experiment. All the proposed methods have been extensively tested, nearly all of them in the United States." Several of the 27 volumes of the CCMC Report are concerned with studies of these actual programs.

Yet the aggregate population covered by programs of organized payment of medical care in 1930 was quite small. In calculating the various sources of U.S. health-related expenditures, the Committee estimated that 14 percent was derived from government (all levels), 5 percent from philanthropy, 2 percent from industry, and all the rest or 79 percent from patients. It did not even include an estimate of funds derived from insurance.

The progress with respect to this, the most contentious, recommendation of the CCMC has been enormous. At the time of the CCMC studies, Blue Cross had not yet taken shape, although the pioneer "group hospitalization plan" of Baylor University Hospital in Dallas, Texas, was described. The voluntary health insurance movement in the United States was promulgated by many social forces, discussed below, but suffice it to say here that by 1981 more than 188 million Americans had insurance for one or more types of health service.[15] This represented 86 percent of the civilian noninstitutional population under 65 years of age and 83 percent of those over 65 (who were mainly protected by public insurance—see below). Hospitalization is the most frequently insured health benefit, but most insured persons also have at least partial protection for the costs of physician's care and various other services.

The financial protection provided by all this insurance coverage is seldom complete, even for hospitalization (which tends to be most fully financed). There are various deductibles, co-payments, maximum amounts, and other limitations that may cause hardship for many people. Because hospital and medical charges are high, insurance premiums are high, and those whose coverage is not shared with or borne by an employer (the great majority are so carried) must pay these premiums regularly themselves. In spite of these and other weaknesses, one must conclude that health insurance on a voluntary basis has fulfilled to a substantial extent the third recommendation of the CCMC. In fact, the development of "health maintenance organizations" (HMOs) and their encouragement by federal subsidies has, in a sense, even gone beyond the recommendations of the CCMC, in their combination of insurance with organization of service.[16] Although HMO enrollment is still relatively small (about 15 million), it has grown at a modest but steady rate.

The organizational and administrative character of U.S. voluntary health insurance, as a whole, admittedly does not correspond to the social spirit of the CCMC recommendation. The largest share of insurance coverage, 55 percent, is through commercial insurance companies, which earn large profits and show little concern for the content or quality of care rendered to policyholders.[17] Experience rating is practiced by nearly all insurance companies, so that high-risk populations, with the greatest health needs, must pay the highest premiums. Competition has forced the nonprofit Blue Cross and Blue Shield insurance plans to do likewise. But with the entrepreneurial setting of American society, could one expect large-scale nongovernmental programs to have developed in any other way?

Beyond voluntary insurance, many other major programs have developed to support the costs of medical care on a "group payment basis," as proposed by the CCMC's third recommendation. The population groups most poorly protected by voluntary health insurance were the aged and the poor. Employment-based coverage terminated when working people retired, and the poor could not afford insurance because they were unemployed or worked in small shops where "fringe benefits" for insurance were not provided. To fill these gaps, after a long political debate, social insurance legislation was enacted to protect the aged and disabled (Medicare), and federal-state tax-supported services were legislated to protect many, though not all, of the poor (Medicaid). In 1980, more than 25 million persons were covered by Medicare and (with some overlap for the poor over age 65) nearly 22 million persons were protected by Medicaid.[18]

Still other population groups have been provided financial protection for medical care since 1930. Out of World War II there grew the program of coverage for military dependents or CHAMPUS (Civilian Health and Medical Program of the Uniformed Services). Veterans' medical benefits, which began following World War I, were greatly extended through a nationwide network of large Veterans Administration hospitals, most of whose patients are being treated for non-service-connected disabilities. American Indians are now served by a special comprehensive medical care program of the U.S. Public Health Service. In all 50 states, worker's compensation now provides medical care protection, as well as partial wage replacement, for persons with work-connected injuries. Apropos of compensation for "wage loss due to illness" called for in the third CCMC recommendation, workers in six states (including the two largest, New York and California) now have statutory insurance for short-term disability, and a much larger number of public and private employees in every state have somewhat equivalent protection through work-connected "sick leave" benefits.

Thus, even without national health insurance, financial protection for medical care costs has become remarkably extensive in America over the last half-century. In the light of extremely high medical and hospital costs at present, the issue of health insurance is now usually discussed in terms of the population *not* protected. As of 1982, some 12 percent of the U.S. population or 28 million people lacked financial access to medical care through either private insurance or public programs.[19] Although a goal of universal coverage was not posed by the CCMC, the magnitude of the problem is clearly very much less than it was in 1930.

COORDINATION OF MEDICAL SERVICES

The fourth recommendation of the CCMC seems less well-defined than the others. It calls for state and local agencies to "evaluate, supplement, and coordinate the medical services of the community" to improve their efficiency and "to stimulate the provision of additional services which are needed." To implement this objective, the Committee recommends the organization of professional groups with lay participants, permanent local coordinating agencies, and state coordinating bodies. Seemingly unrelated is a proposal for much more rigorous state and federal drug control legislation.

Judgment on achievements with respect to this recommendation can hardly be optimistic. The fragmentation and pluralism of the American health care system have remained with us. Countless coordinating councils have been formed in local communities and at the state level, often focused on special problems, such as care of the aged, mental illness, child health, or accident prevention. Their impacts have usually been slight and short-lived. It is especially unfortunate that state and local health departments, which would seem most appropriate for this role, have not played it—nor was this even recommended by the CCMC.

Regarding the specific recommendation on drug regulation, one can be more positive. The federal legislation on "food and drug control" of 1939, and the further amendments to this law of 1962, have provided vastly stronger protection to drug consumers than prevailed in 1930. The manufacture of drugs, as well as their labeling, advertising, and sale, are now subject to controls that are quite effective in protecting the population from harm or from fraud.

The fourth recommendation speaks also of "coordination of urban and rural facilities," which calls to mind the objectives of the Hill-Burton Act of 1946, with its "master plans" for hospital construction in each state, and the Regional Medical Program legislation of 1965, with its provision for the extension of urban medical technology to rural hospitals. Neither of these legislative measures, however, has been very successful in achieving effective professional relationships among the health facilities in a region.[20]

Perhaps the social action closest to the import of the fourth CCMC recommendation was the legislation of 1966 on Comprehensive Health Planning and its follow-up law of 1974 (the National Health Planning and Resource Development Act), establishing a nationwide network of "health systems agencies." In their objectives, both these measures called for assessment of community health needs, coordination of programs, and the stimulation of actions to respond to unmet needs. Except for limited impacts on the hospital bed supply in communities, however, to restrict overbuilding, few would claim that either of these laws achieved its objectives.[21] Under the Reagan administration, furthermore, these planning efforts at the local level have been greatly eroded, leaving mainly skeleton agencies at the state level.

BASIC EDUCATIONAL IMPROVEMENTS

The fifth recommendation of the CCMC calls for strengthening the social content of the education of physicians and other health professionals, as well as training health administrators. In 1930, American medical education was still very much under the influence of the Flexner Report, with its great emphasis on basic sciences and advanced technology; medical schools showed little concern for preventive or social concepts. The Committee stated also that "the real needs of the people call for three to five times as many well-trained general practitioners as specialists, and most schools, therefore, should concentrate their energies on producing well-qualified general practitioners." Greater opportunities for high-grade postgraduate education were also called for.

Pharmaceutical education, it was recommended, should emphasize the "pharmacist's responsibility for public health and safety." Nursing education should be revised to "produce socially-minded nurses, with a preparation basic to all types of nursing service" (i.e., not only in hospitals, but in community posts). "Nursing attendants" or auxiliary nurses, who would work under supervision, should also be trained. Furthermore, nurse-midwives should be trained and licensed to handle all normal deliveries. Finally, to manage hospitals and clinics administrators should be trained, who "can understand and integrate the various professional, economic, and social factors involved."

Assessing the progress made since 1930 on the fifth recommendation gives a somewhat mixed but generally positive picture. In medical education, preventive and social concepts have certainly received greater attention, either as special disciplines or as aspects of clinical subjects.[22] Among the 126 medical schools in the nation, virtually all now offer some instruction in the main characteristics of disease in populations (epidemiology), although probably not more than half have well-developed departments of preventive medicine, community health, or the social dimensions of medicine identified by other terms. A stronger academic response has been shown to the need for greater emphasis on training well-qualified general practitioners. By the late 1960s, a worldwide reaction to excessive specialization had set in, and a new appreciation developed for the well-rounded and sensitive family doctor. In 1969, a formal specialty qualification was established in the United States for "family practice," and most medical schools set up new departments, or new subdivisions of traditional departments, in this field.[23] Often family practice was combined with community health—adding an attractive clinical flavor to this population-oriented field, but also diminishing the social character of such a combined department's teaching.

In pharmacy education, about one-third of the nation's 72 schools were offering instruction on the social aspects of the field in 1972, and by 1980 this proportion was doubtless higher.[24] With the virtual disappearance of individual drug-compounding in pharmacies, the modern pharmacist has time to play a much larger health role in communities, particularly in the health education of clients.

The entire field of nursing education has undergone enormous changes since 1930. The hospital-based nursing school has been gradually replaced by educational programs in academic settings—both universities and junior colleges—where greater attention is given to community nursing functions.[25] Also, the training of "nursing attendants" or vocational nurses (as they are now usually called) has greatly expanded, and these personnel are now licensed by almost all states. Only in the field of nurse-midwifery has the progress been limited; while the training programs for nurse-midwives have increased, by 1982 only 1.8 percent of deliveries in the nation were handled by midwives.[26]

Regarding the education of hospital and clinic administrators, the recommendations of the Committee have been more than fulfilled. In 1934, two years after publication of the CCMC Final Report, the first university-based program of training for hospital administration was established at the University of Chicago. Since then, the number of such training programs—now usually defined more broadly as "health service administration"—has increased to more than 50.[27] Most of these are associated with university schools of business or public administration or of management, but several are departments within schools of public health. Especially noteworthy has been the steadily broadened academic content of these programs, with the objective of preparing health care administrators to understand the wider community role of their institutions.[28]

Finally, it may be noted that in all the health care professions, not only in medicine and dentistry (as proposed by the Committee), postgraduate and continuing education has been greatly expanded. Professional schools, associations, voluntary health agencies, hospitals, and other entitites offer an endless stream of symposia and courses on new developments in every branch of health science. Many hospitals have appointed part-time or full-time "directors of continuing education" to assure the quality of their programs. Most U.S. states now require that a certain number of hours of continuing education be attended each year by various health professionals, for maintenance of their licensure or registration.[29] Here again, developments have probably surpassed the recommendations of the CCMC.

CAUSES OF PROGRESS

In summary, one may conclude that four of the five recommendations of the CCMC have *in large measure* been fulfilled. Only the fourth recommendation, on the coordination of the highly pluralistic American health care system, has shown little fulfillment, although the actions taken toward national health planning—while largely aborted in recent years—may well serve as precursors to more effective coordination in the future. With respect to the organization of medical services, the strengthening of public health, group payment, and educational improvements, the progress has been substantial—exceeding in several respects the advocacy of the Committee.

This is not to say that the several health system developments have corresponded precisely to the types of action proposed by the Committee. New patterns of health care organization and financing have, after all, had to reflect the balance of social forces at play in American society—a balance that one could hardly expect the most insightful group of scholars and leaders to anticipate. But the essential aims of the major recommendations, and the many subsidiary proposals for implementation, have been achieved to a remarkably large extent.

This positive assessment does not mean, of course, that the changes can be attributed solely or even mainly to the recommendations of the CCMC. Countless developments in society and in technology have been responsible for the evolution of the American health services. The great economic Depression of the 1930s was just beginning, as the Committee was drawing up its final report. American capitalism was facing a crisis greater than any it had ever experienced before, and a whole succession of social reforms, the New Deal, was generated. The organized labor movement, which had been quite weak, acquired much greater strength. Collective bargaining between labor and management gave rise to the "fringe benefit"—often the payment of health insurance premiums. The U.S. economy became increasingly industrialized and the population urbanized. Science and technology, of course, expanded enormously, leading to greater medical benefits and also higher costs. World War II and the Atlantic Charter generated demands for a better postwar life, reflected most dramatically in the British National Health Service. The notion that modern medical science could accomplish wonders, if only it were made available to people needing it, made health care a political issue. Better living conditions and preventive measures greatly reduced the infectious diseases of childhood, changed the age-composition of the population, and heightened vastly the importance of the chronic disorders of later life, which required long-term and costly medical care.

These were only the more important developments shaping the U.S. health care system between 1930 and 1980. The impact of a body of health services research—even of the monumental proportions of the CCMC—must be considered faint by comparison. But is it even reasonable to look upon health services research as a *cause* of social change?

The contributions of the CCMC, in my opinion, illustrate very well the proper function of health services research (HSR). If HSR is oriented to the clarification of problems in the health care system, if it poses the "right questions" so that the findings point to policy responses, then its contribution to improvement of the health care system in any country can be very great. In effect, HSR findings can serve as instruments for helping to achieve social change. Modification of the status quo in health or any other field invariably entails controversy. Findings like those of the CCMC provide invaluable ammunition for the advocates of changes needed for the solution of problems.

A central finding of the CCMC, for example, was the highly uneven incidence of illness. In any one year, the Committee found, a small fraction of the people bear the great bulk of the costs. The obvious solution was to spread health care costs over groups of people and over periods of time—the essential principle of insurance. But in 1930, the application of insurance to medical costs was a strange and fearful idea. The American Medical Association was not the only group to view it with alarm. CCMC data proved to be extremely valuable in showing the eminently good sense of health insurance financing.

Another key finding of the CCMC was that the lower income groups suffered a greater burden of illness, but they received lesser rates of all types of medical care than the well-to-do. Inequities might be tolerated in clothing or housing or transportation, but no social or political leader could defend such inequities in the treatment of a sick child or woman or man. Again, the findings of the CCMC, and many more HSR efforts that followed, were effective tools for achieving greater equity in health services.

Accomplishments on the whole issue of health care equity have been particularly impressive. Based on its nationwide survey in 1928–1931, the CCMC found the rate of contacts with physicians and the rate of hospitalizations to vary directly with family income. The figures are shown in Table 7.1. Fifty years later, the corresponding rates of health services found in a nation-wide survey are shown in Table 7.2. While there are small differences in the definitions and methodology for the two periods, the essential changes are clear and dramatic. In 1928–1931, the lowest income groups had the lowest rate of contacts with physicians and the lowest rate of hospital admissions, while the highest income groups had the highest such rates. In 1981, these rates of medical care utilization had greatly increased for all income groups. More significant, the relationships between lower and higher income groups were completely reversed. Data not given here show that in both periods the volume of sickness and disability was greater among the poor. The response of the health care system in 1930 was perverse—opposite to the extent of health needs. By 1981, social actions had been taken to result in rates of medical care generally appropriate to the differential needs; low-income groups with more sickness received more medical care and high-income groups with less sickness received less care. This is not to imply that perfect equity has been attained, but the trends are clearly in that direction.

Table 7.1.   Medical Care and Family Income, United States 1928–1931

Family Income	Physician Contacts per Person per Year	Hospital Cases per 1000 Persons per Year
1. Lowest	1.9	59.4
2.	2.0	52.4
3.	2.3	59.4
4.	2.7	63.1
5.	3.6	79.3
6. Highest	4.7	98.0

Source: Committee on the Costs of Medical Care, *Medical Care for the American People—Final Report,* 1932, p. 8.

Table 7.2.   Medical Care and Family Income, United States, 1981

Family Income	Physician Contacts per Person per Year	Hospital Cases per 1000 Persons per Year
1. Lowest	5.6	165.1
2.	4.9	137.5
3.	4.5	124.5
4.	4.5	119.8
5. Highest	4.4	104.6

Source: U.S. National Center for Health Statistics, *Health—United States, 1983*, pp. 137, 149.

NATIONAL HEALTH INSURANCE

If so much progress has occurred in the American health care system—supported by the powerful findings of the CCMC—why then has national health insurance not been enacted? After all, the National Health Conference of 1938 attempted to bring about "completion" of the Social Security Act of 1935, with addition of social insurance provisions for medical care. For 40 years since 1939, legislative proposals for national health insurance were introduced into Congress. I. S. Falk played a role at almost every step of the way. He and many others believed that, with proper universal economic support for health services, most of the other changes needed in the health care system could be rapidly attained.

The wisdom of hindsight suggests that the very progress we have reviewed in American health services has served, in many ways, to obstruct the attainment of national health insurance. The robust growth of voluntary health insurance, despite all its inadequacies, has still met a great deal of the need and has blunted the demands for government-sponsored universal coverage. This has applied especially to organized union labor, which might have been the strongest force for national political action but was, at the same time, the population sector best protected by voluntary insurance plans. And paradoxically, it was the very prominence of public debate on national insurance that stimulated private insurance carriers to double their efforts for enrollment of people. "If private insurance does not do the job," they thought, "government will take over."

Later, in the 1960s, when the weakness of private health insurance in protecting the aged and the poor became glaring, Medicare and Medicaid came to the rescue. The end of the Roosevelt and Truman years, with the election of Eisenhower in 1952, led to defeatism about universal insurance coverage and to the "tactical retreat" (as expressed by I. S. Falk) that culminated in Medicare and Medicaid. Attaining enactment of even these laws, however, meant "compromise with the private insurance industry, with the medical and hospital providers, and with state and local welfare agencies [which] was potentially disastrous."[30] A high price, in escalating health care costs, was paid for this patchwork legislation, even though—like voluntary insurance—it neutralized further social pressures for national health insurance.

Other factors responsible for the failure of national health insurance to be enacted may be gleaned from comparison with Europe, where national public action was taken everywhere. In America there was no Labor Party nor Social Democratic Party, such as plays a key political role in virtually every country of Europe. Voluntary insurance preceded public legislation in all European countries, but these insurance funds were tied to labor groups, political groups, religious groups—not to health care providers and commercial companies, as in America. The whole spirit of entrepreneurialism that characterized the United States embodied also a deep aversion to government. Unlike Europe, the world of American hospitals was dominated by nongovernmental institutions, and the medical profession was dominated by conservative high-income specialists rather than moderate-income general practitioners.[31]

Next to these influences, the frontal opposition to national health insurance by the American Medical Association probably played a relatively minor part. (One may recall that the intense AMA opposition to Medicare in the 1960s was not effective.) The very opposition of the AMA to national insurance, in fact, served to mollify the attitudes of medical societies toward other health measures, such as the Hill-Burton hospital construction program, subsidy of medical research, or federal grants to the states for strengthening public health programs. Much of the progress in the health care system reviewed above was, in a sense, made in response to the "threat value" of the national health insurance legislative debate.

CURRENT ISSUES

The prominent issues of national discussion about the health care system in the 1980s are very different from those of previous years—from issues of the 1970s, let alone the decades back to 1930. Concern for access to care and equity may still win the attention of socially minded health workers, but in most social debate on the health care system, the discussion is now dominated by costs. Many voices of conservatism point an accusing finger at various social programs as responsible for the medical care cost escalation. They forget that the largest of such programs, Medicare and Medicaid, were designed—in order to assure their enactment—with very meager regulatory constraints. (It has been said that the Medicare Law was passed by its friends, but written by its enemies.) They call for a return to the free market and competition as the path to cost containment, overlooking the basic inapplicability of market principles to the medical care process.[32] With the rejection by many of government intervention and even voluntary nonprofit sponsorship, the management of hospitals and nursing homes has come increasingly under the control of private for-profit corporations.[33]

Yet in the very effort to control costs, increasing attention is being drawn to health maintenance organizations, despite the long history of opposition to their essential principle—health insurance linked to group medical practice. In fact, in his last major paper on the CCMC, I. S. Falk speaks of the combination of insurance with "organized comprehensive nonprofit group practice" as the "centerpiece" of CCMC recommendations—really a blend of the first and the third recommendations.[30] Falk saw the HMO as the brightest hope on the horizon of medical care development in America which, in so many respects, he characterized as a discouraging and "mournful tale."

In spite of the currently entrepreneurial character of the U.S. health care system, the story of the 50 years since the CCMC has been mainly one of definite progress toward equity and efficiency—progress through greater organization of health services (to enhance their quality and efficiency), through the extension of preventive services (under public health and other auspices), through increasing social support of health care costs (extending their equitable distribution), and through broadened education of all types of health manpower.[34] Only with respect to the CCMC recommendation on greater "coordination of medical service" has the deep-seated attribute of American pluralism prevailed, so that the overall system of health care is probably more fragmented than ever.

The ultimate test of progress in a health care system is the general health status of the people. Life expectancy at birth in the United States has risen from 47.3 years in 1900 to 74.5 years in 1982. Even at age 65 years, in 1900 the average American could expect to live another 11.9 years, compared with an expectation of 16.8 additional years in 1982. Infant mortality declined from 29.2 per 1000 live births in 1950 to 11.2 in 1982. Many social and environmental factors, of course, influence mortality rates, but there is no doubt that health services, preventive and therapeutic, play a significant part. The quality of life has also been improved by modern medical care and rehabilitation. National health expenditures have risen from 3.5 percent of gross national product in 1929 to 10.5 percent of a much larger GNP in 1982; this amounted to an expenditure of $29 per capita in 1929 and $1365 per capita in 1982. There is much evidence of waste and inefficiency in these large expenditures, but one can hardly deny that the health care system trends over this half-century have constituted progress. The work of I. S. Falk and the Committee on the Costs of Medical Care have contributed significantly to that progress.

REFERENCES

1. Hirshfield D: The Lost Reform: The Campaign for Compulsory Health Insurance in the United States from 1932 to 1943. Cambridge: Harvard University Press, 1970.
2. This account of Falk's life is drawn largely from an essay by R. Joseph Anderson, Nancy Robertson, Alan Hoffman, and Sharon Laist, introducing the collection of "Isadore S. Falk Papers" in the Yale University, Sterling Memorial Library, Manuscripts and Archives. They constitute Manuscript Group Number 1039 of the "Contemporary Medical Care and Health Policy Collection," September 1981, New Haven, Conn.
3. U.S. Senate, Committee on Finance: Comparison of Major Features of Health Insurance Proposals. Washington, DC: GPO 1979.
4. Iggers GG: Historicism. In: Wiener PP (Ed): Dictionary of the History of Ideas. New York: C Scribner's, 1973; 2:456–464.
5. Fox DM: The decline of historicism: The case of compulsory health insurance in the United States. *Bull History Med,* 1983; 57:596–610.
6. Falk IS: The Committee on the Costs of Medical Care—25 years of progress. Am J Public Health, August 1958; 48:979–1002.
7. Committee on the Costs of Medical Care: Medical Care for the American People: The Final Report of the Committee. Chicago: University of Chicago Press, 1932; 104–144.
8. Donaledion A, Axelrod SJ, Wyszewianski L: Medical Care Chartbook (7th ed). Ann Arbor, Mich: Health Administration Press, 1980; 166.
9. Kahn HS, Orris P: The emerging role of salaried physicians: An organizational proposal. J Public Health Policy September 1982; 3:284–292.

10. Roemer MI: Ambulatory Health Services in America. Rockville, Md: Aspen Systems Corp., 1981; 128–132.
11. Roemer MI: Ambulatory Health Services in America. Rockville, Md: Aspen Systems Corp., 1981; 139–169.
12. Roemer MI, Friedman JW: Doctors in Hospitals: Medical Staff Organization and Hospital Performance. Baltimore: Johns Hopkins Press, 1971.
13. Roemer MI: The politics of public health in the United States. In: Litman TJ, Robins LS (Eds): Health Politics and Policy. New York: Wiley, 1984; 261–273.
14. US Public Health Services: Healthy People: The Surgeon General's Report on Health Promotion and Disease Prevention. Washington, DC: Department of Health, Education and Welfare, 1979.
15. Health Insurance Association of America: Source Book of Health Insurance Data 1982–1983, Washington, DC: 1983.
16. Luft HS: Health Maintenance Organizations: Dimensions of Performance. New York: Wiley, 1981.
17. Hetherington RW, Hopkins CE, Roemer MI: Health Insurance Plans: Promise and Performance. New York: Wiley, 1975.
18. US Social Security Administration: Social Security Bulletin: Annual Statistical Supplement, 1982, 200–219.
19. Robert Wood Johnson Foundation: Special Report: Updated Report on Access to Health Care for the American People, Number One, 1983.
20. Bodenheimer TS: Regional medical programs: No road to regionalization. Med Care Rev December 1969; 26:1125–1166.
21. Shonick W: Health planning. In: Last JM (Ed): Maxcy-Rosenau Public Health and Preventive Medicine (12th ed). New York: Appleton, Century, Crofts, in press.
22. Deuschle KW, Eberson F: Community medicine comes of age. J Med Educ December 1968; 43:1229–1237.
23. Silberstein EB, Scott CJ: An evaluation of undergraduate family care programs. J Community Health 1978; 3:369–379.
24. Wertheimer AI, Smith MC: Pharmacy Practice—Social and Behavioral Aspects. Baltimore: University Park Press, 1974; xiii.
25. Kalisch PA, Kalisch BJ: The Advance of American Nursing. Boston: Little, Brown, 1978.
26. Adams CJ: Nurse-Midwifery Practice in the United States, 1982. Am J Public Health November 1984; 74:1267–1270.
27. Association of University Programs of Health Administration: Health Services Administration Education 1983–85. Washington, DC: 1982.
28. Commission on Education for Health Administration: Report (2 volumes). Ann Arbor, Mich: Health Administration Press, 1975.
29. Gaumer GL: Regulating health personnel: A review of the empirical literature. Milbank Mem Fund Q Summer 1984; 62:380–416.
30. Falk IS: Some lessons from the fifty years since the CCMC Final Report, 1932. J Public Health Policy June 1983; 4:135–161.
31. Roemer MI, Roemer RJ: Health Care Systems and Comparative Manpower Policies. New York: Marcel Dekker, 1981; 284.

32. Roemer MI: Market failure and health care policy. J Public Health Policy December 1982; 3:419–431.
33. Relman AS: The new medical-industrial complex. N Engl J Med 1980; 303:963–970.
34. Roemer MI: An Introduction to the U.S. Health Care System. New York: Springer, 1982; 111–124.

Chapter **8**

Medical Ethics and Education for Social Responsibility

Forty years ago Henry Sigerist delivered the Terry Lectures at Yale, under the title *Medicine and Human Welfare*. With elegant simplicity he traced the historical development of society's concepts of disease, of health, and of the role of the physician. In concluding the last lecture, he said:

> The scope of medicine has indeed broadened. . . . No longer a shaman, priest, craftsman, or cleric, [the physician] must be more than a mere scientist. We begin to perceive the outline of a new physician. Scientist and social worker, prepared to cooperate in teamwork and in close touch with the people he serves; a friend and leader, he will direct all his efforts toward the prevention of disease and become a therapist when prevention has broken down—the social physician protecting the people and guiding them to a healthier and happier life.[1]

Like so much of Sigerist's writing, these words were meant to be partly a forecast based on past historical trends, and partly an inspirational call to work toward future goals.

RESPONSIBILITY TO THE INDIVIDUAL PATIENT

For centuries, society has defined the obligations of the physician solely in terms of his responsibilities to individual patients. Every medical student is familiar with the Code of Hammurabi, 2000 B.C., under which

149

the Babylonian surgeon was rewarded—or indeed punished—for the results of his efforts, depending on their outcome and the social status of the patient. The Hippocratic oath, despite its mysterious origins, is still sworn to by new medical graduates—perhaps mainly to forge a link with an ancient calling; yet its affirmations speak only of the doctor's maintenance of honorable relations with each patient and of devotion to his teacher.

Medical licensure had its beginnings in the Middle Ages, and was linked to the standard of competence formulated by the newly founded universities. In 1140, the Norman king Roger decreed:

> Who, from now on, wishes to practice medicine, has to present himself before our officials and examiners, in order to pass their judgment . . . In this way we are taking care that our subjects are not endangered by the inexperience of the physicians. Nobody dare practice medicine unless he has been found fit by the convention of the Salernitan masters.

Aside from some generalities about good moral character, little more is to be found in the medical licensure laws of today. In the main, they are more specific about the required educational preparation and the examinations to be passed. One searches in vain for provisions in the licensure laws about obligations of doctors to serve people in need, to cooperate with public authorities on the prevention of disease, always to put the patient's welfare above pecuniary gain, or any other doctrine defining medicine's social responsibilities.

Other formal influences on medical behavior arose not under law, but through the self-disciplinary rules formulated within the medical profession itself. With the rise of industrialism and mercantilism in the late eighteenth century, physicians inevitably became small businessmen. The problems emerging were those associated with the marketplace—"unfair practices" that could occur when physicians competed for patients.

In response, societies of physicians—first in Europe, then in America and elsewhere—developed codes of ethics. These called for "professional conduct" in the relationship between physicians and patients and among physicians. The early nineteenth-century code in America even spoke of "the duty of physicians to be ever vigilant for the welfare of the community."

Deeds, of course, speak louder than words. Whatever may have been the lofty counsel of the ethical codes of physicians, we can learn more about the evolution of a professional sense of social responsibility—and the trials and tribulations along the way—by examining the actual relationships of physicians to the principal components of health care systems.

RELATIONS TO PUBLIC HEALTH MEASURES

The important leadership in the origins of the public health movement in England came, not from a physician, but from Edwin Chadwick—a wealthy public-spirited citizen of Lancashire—who reported in 1842 on the *Sanitary Conditions of the Labouring Population of Great Britain*. Likewise, the first state public health agency in America resulted from the zealous efforts of a Boston bookseller, Lemuel Shattuck. In later times socially oriented physicians, among them Edward Trudeau, Herman Biggs, and Thomas Parran, gave crucial leadership in other sectors of public health; but these were courageous men, not at all representative of their contemporaries in the medical profession.

Sixty years ago the posture of the main body of the medical profession in America toward public health advances was well illustrated by its reactions to the Sheppard-Towner Act of 1921; this was the first legislation calling for federal grants to the states in order to help them establish preventively oriented maternal and child health clinics. In the aftermath of the Women's Suffrage Amendment to the Constitution in 1920, opposition to an "Act for the promotion of the welfare of maternity and infancy" could hardly be strong, but by 1926 the American Medical Association had hardened its stand. Outright opposition was mounted in every state, and by 1929 the program had been destroyed. Not until the bleak Depression of the 1930s were federal grants to the states for maternal and child health and for other public health purposes resumed, in the Social Security Act of 1935. One might cite many more public health actions that could proceed only after overcoming the opposition of private doctors. Moreover, it is still not easy to recruit physicians for service in maternal and child health and other public health clinics that serve essentially low-income families.

ATTITUDES TOWARD SOCIAL FINANCING OF MEDICAL CARE

The attitude of the medical profession as a whole toward social measures to increase the economic access of patients to medical care has ranged from indifferent to cool to bitterly hostile. In early nineteenth-century Europe, when mutual aid funds were formed to help low-income people cope with the economic burden of sickness (wage loss) and medical care, the initiative was taken by workers. Doctors not flourishing with a carriage trade were glad to have these regular clients. After 1870, the same was true in the United States, where mutual benefit associations were founded, largely by European immigrant workers.

The opposition of the American medical profession to the development of any type of insurance for medical care is an especially long saga. Voluntary "Blue Cross" insurance plans to pay for hospitalization were attacked as "half-baked schemes." Proposals for national health insurance legislation, both before and since the Second World War, have been condemned with particular rancor as "socialized medicine." Even when health insurance coverage was to be restricted to elderly pensioners in the 1960s, medical opposition continued. With overwhelming popular support, however, "Medicare" for the aged was enacted in 1965. Soon after this program started, medical and hospital costs rose so rapidly that numerous social controls had to be imposed, including the establishment of a federal office on fraud and abuse.

Lest medical opposition to the social financing of health care be regarded as a peculiarly American phenomenon, one need only be reminded of the perennial conflicts between physicians and social insurance authorities in Australia, France, Germany, Great Britain, Japan, and elsewhere. Doctors have not refrained from "strikes," or outright withholding of services from patients, in opposing the implementation of health insurance laws duly enacted by parliamentary bodies. Such action was threatened by the British Medical Association shortly before the effective date of the British National Health Service in 1948. Doctors in Saskatchewan, Canada, actually withheld all except emergency services for 23 days after the 1962 opening date of the Medical Care Insurance program in that province. Yet within six years legislation was enacted to cover all of Canada with similar services. Between 1960 and 1968, no fewer than 16 doctor strikes occurred in seven European countries, as part of medical resistance to health insurance operations.[2]

MEDICAL EDUCATION AND PHYSICIAN SUPPLY

In America in the late nineteenth century, scientific advances were very rapid, but doctors were being trained at scores of mediocre schools. Abraham Flexner, educator but not physician, was appointed by the Carnegie Foundation to survey the situation, and his famous report of 1910 had enormous impact. The quality of medical education became vastly improved, both in its scientific content and in the use of full-time teachers.[3] Through a system of "grading" schools, the substandard ones were gradually eliminated. Leaders of the medical profession embraced the report, and the American Medical Association participated in the grading program.

But there was another side to the impact of the Flexner report. Medical education became highly technological, with little room for teaching about medicine's ultimately social role.[4] And questions about the numbers and types of doctors necessary to meet the population's health needs were not even posed.

As was to be expected, the doctor-to-population ratio in the United States declined for 20 years after the Flexner report; then, from 1930 to 1960, the output of doctors barely kept up with population growth. Meanwhile, the steadily rising demands for medical care—due to greater public education, purchasing power, and other factors—could be handled only through vastly expanded training of nurses and other health personnel.[5] With federal subsidies of medical schools, the doctor-to-population ratio began to improve about 1960, but this was achieved only after overcoming the long resistance to such subsidies from the private medical profession. Clarification of the nation's need for more doctors came not from the medical profession, but from the U.S. Public Health Service—particularly through the work of one of its most courageous leaders, Dr. Joseph W. Mountin.[6]

The enormous growth of medical specialization (currently about 85 percent of practicing doctors in the United States are specialists), with a resultant steep decline in the number of generalists and primary care doctors, is another long-term consequence of the policies characterizing the post-Flexner era in American medicine. The trend has been reflected in rising problems of patient access to primary care and spiraling demands on hospital emergency departments. The extremely high proportion of surgeons and surgical specialties in the United States (relative to other countries) has undoubtedly led to excessive rates of surgical operations. It has also probably contributed to the avalanche of medical malpractice suits, of a magnitude not seen in any other country.

What has been the response of the American medical profession to these problems? Has it been to recommend actions that would reduce the training of specialists and increase the output of primary care doctors? Not at all. It has been to encourage the training of various doctor-substitutes, known as "physician assistants" and "nurse practitioners."[7] These personnel are intended to serve principally the poor in inner-city slums and the rural areas, where primary care shortages have been very critical. By contrast, other industrialized countries—where specialization has developed to a reasonable degree and where close to half the doctors are engaged in primary care—have rejected these lesser trained personnel for primary care; instead, they have emphasized the further strengthening of general medical practice.[8] The USSR slowed up the training of *feldshers* some years ago, when its supply of physicians was deemed adequate. On the other hand, most European countries use trained midwives for normal deliveries—yielding a great saving of physician manpower. Yet, in spite of the superior maternal mortality record of these countries, most American obstetricians have opposed these effective health personnel, for reasons that are not hard to guess.

A more socially sound response to the American deficiencies in primary care medicine has come from the U.S. Congress, which has provided financial inducement to increase residency training in primary care. After many years of resistance from the dominant body of specialists in the American profession, a "specialty" status for family practice was established in 1969, in order to enhance the social standing and potential earnings of medical generalists.

ENTREPRENEURSHIP IN MEDICINE— A WORLDWIDE PHENOMENON

This may be enough information to support the conclusion that medicine in recent decades has become seriously corrupted by a spirit of entrepreneurship. The poignant image of the devoted horse-and-buggy doctor of a century ago may or may not have been as generally valid as one might be led to believe. But in the current era, the lofty medical traditions of human service have clearly become eroded by essentially commercial objectives. Although the discussion here has been mainly concerned with the American setting—and commercialized medicine is probably more extreme in that bastion of free enterprise than elsewhere—the problem is by no means limited to the United States.

In Germany, where the social insurance concept was first applied to medical care in the 1880s, physician abuse of the fee system of remuneration has long been a problem.[9] More than 85 percent of the West German population is now covered by the mandatory insurance program, but there are frequent complaints that the minority of private or voluntarily insured patients are treated more solicitously than the socially insured. Unwarranted multiplication of office visits for minor illness has long been a widely recognized abuse in Japan's health insurance system. In the Belgian health insurance system, medical fees are frequently inflated beyond the officially approved level, and the rate of home calls, compared with office visits, is inordinately high because the former command larger insurance fees.[10]

The retention of fee-for-service payment of doctors under social insurance programs, in order to satisfy the medical profession, presents a constant regulatory challenge to public authorities. In Canada, where each of the 10 provinces administers its own scheme, a whole spectrum of disciplinary strategies has been found necessary. Salaried remuneration of doctors, frequently used for hospital specialists, is associated with other abuses. In Sweden, excessive private practice after official hours caused such serious inequities that the government was forced to ban this "privilege" in 1972, a policy adopted soon thereafter by Norway. In the British National Health Service, limited private practice by salaried hospital consultants has long been allowed, despite the inequities it causes; under the current British government, these inequities are being aggravated through encouraging the sale of personal insurance to facilitate the purchase of private service by greater numbers of affluent people, who can afford to pay twice.

In Australia, the highly political private medical profession played a significant role in destroying an entire national health insurance program that had been legislated in 1974. The Australian Medical Association, along with the private insurance industry and others, obstructed the program's implementation sufficiently to lead to a political crisis. By 1979, the Australian National Health Insurance program of 1974 had been completely dismantled.[11]

Physician abuse and obstruction of social financing programs, designed to increase the equitable access of people to medical care, are not limited to the affluent industrial countries, but are widespread throughout the developing world. In Latin America, for example, physicians serving in a public program part-time (three or four hours a day) frequently cut corners in their official duties in order to extend their time in private practice. In governmental health services on every continent, doctors seeing patients hastily in public clinics advise some of them that more solicitous care would be available in the doctor's private office.

Entrepreneurship is found even in the medical services of the socialist countries. Publicly financed health care has been developed to a very high level in the Soviet Union and other socialist countries, but private practice has never been banned, and people may seek private care from a doctor after his official duty hours. In Poland, this pattern has been institutionalized through so-called medical cooperatives, in which doctors may work up to two hours a day after their public service. The fees are officially regulated, but they must, of course, be paid by the patient privately.[12]

PRESSURES TOWARD SOCIALLY ORIENTED MEDICAL BEHAVIOR

This recitation about medical behavior in the health care systems of America and throughout the world—behavior so often contrary to the best interests of patients, particularly the least fortunate members of any society—is surely enough to suggest the contours of a problem not merely in personal morality but in the social ethics of medicine. It is not so much the behavior of the doctor to the individual patient or the relationship of one doctor to another that is involved: it is the attitude, the practices, and the policies of doctors toward the total population that are involved or, more accurately, the medical profession's sense of social responsibility.

In spite of all the medical opposition to change in national health systems, the quality and distribution of health services have been improved in most countries. Social insurance programs have removed economic barriers to medical care for millions of people. Community health centers or posts with trained personnel have extended health services to large rural populations. In many countries, drugs are regulated and hospitals are inspected in order to uphold standards and protect patients. These advances, however, have been achieved mainly because of pressure from the public and the leadership of nonmedical men and women.

Is it not reasonable to inquire why so much of the influence for achieving social equity, altruism, and idealism has arisen outside the medical profession, not within it? Why has so much social effort been required to counteract entrepreneurial behavior by physicians, to impose regulation and disciplinary measures to compel medical performance that is more beneficial for patients? The answer really calls for another question: Why should one expect the physician to behave according to values different from those that prevail in the society around him?

The principal guiding ethos of most of the world for several hundred years has been private profit—personal self-interest. But this has not been the *only* precept on which modern societies have been built. At the same time there have been countless movements for community welfare, for social solidarity to protect the least fortunate.[13] In part the motivation has come from religion, from the belief that kindness and mercy bring rewards to the giver as well as the receiver; and in part it has come from the calculated efforts of each social order to maintain its stability, to resist overthrow by those who are discontented and enraged about their suffering. As Henry Sigerist pointed out, social security was pioneered by the conservative German Chancellor Bismarck not to launch a revolution but to prevent one.

Whichever philosophical rationale for humanitarianism one may prefer, the challenge to medical ethics is to influence physician behavior in the direction of enhancing concern for the well-being of the greatest proportion of people. Admittedly, behavior is bound to be influenced more by social circumstances than by formal teaching: a cooperative community setting will generate more cooperative behavior than a competitive jungle, regardless of moralistic litanies. Yet, insofar as moral teachings can influence behavior, what should they be? What should be included in a code of medical ethics clearly oriented toward social responsibility?

TOWARD A SOCIAL ETHICS
OF MEDICINE

In the light of medicine's long historical development toward a goal of equity, I would suggest that a modern code of ethics should put its major emphasis on the doctor's social responsibilities. I do not imply abandonment of long-established precepts for a virtuous doctor–patient relationship, such as doing the patient no harm, respecting individual dignity, and protecting the confidentiality of medical communication. But far too many treatises on medical ethics, even in modern times, are limited to issues of this sort, along with precepts on sexuality, contraception, sterilization, and abortion, which are essentially part of the doctrine of particular religious creeds.

All this is not to deny the need for sound ethical practices to govern the doctor's relationship to individual patients. In these days of elaborate life-support systems for dying patients, of high-technology incubators to maintain alive extremely small and handicapped infants, of artificial kidney machines and transplanted hearts, and much more, ethical decisions are faced every day. The question often comes to "how much should be spent (from limited resources) to keep a certain patient alive?" This difficult issue arises most often in hospitals, and in many of them Hospital Ethics Committees have been established to bear the responsibility for the decision. Individual cases of this type are dramatic, and are all too often reported in the daily press, but the larger ethical questions on provision of health care to populations remain the most important.

Worldwide developments toward achieving equity in health care, however, are seldom communicated to students in medical school. The post-Flexner era in American medical education, as noted earlier, has turned out mainly specialized technologists with little sensitivity to medicine's social role. Similar concepts have come to dominate medical education in most other countries.[14] What can be done to launch another Flexnerian revolution for training in the social, as well as the technical, functions of the doctor?

Following the revelations about the brutal behavior of physicians in Nazi Germany, who conducted lethal experiments on human beings, the world medical community established principles that might prevent repetition of such atrocities. These were set forth in the Declaration of Helsinki on Biomedical Research Involving Human Subjects. In the same spirit, observation of worldwide social trends in health care, along with recognition of the many problems encountered in attempting to achieve health care equity, should lead to the formulation of a new Ethical Code on Medicine's Social Responsibility.

From the streamlined Code of Ethics formulated by the World Medical Association in 1948 in its Declaration of Geneva, I would retain only the opening clause: "I solemnly pledge myself to consecrate my life to the service of humanity."[15] The pledges to practice the profession with dignity, to respect one's teachers, to regard other physicians as brothers, and so on, would find little justification in a code on social responsibility. In their place I would add the following:

- I will do whatever I can to help my patient and the whole community to prevent disease or injury and to maintain good health.
- I will respect the dignity of all persons, serving them in accordance with their health needs, irrespective of their personal status or the pecuniary rewards involved.
- Realizing the greater health problems of the poor, I will make a special effort to respond to their needs.
- Conscious always that the cost of health care is borne by the people, I will do nothing wasteful or without justification.
- In spite of the attractions of certain localities, I will serve the people where they live and work, wherever my skills are most needed.
- I will serve cooperatively with other health workers, in the interests of effective provision of health service.
- I will cooperate with public authorities in the implementation of health legislation that reflects the democratic decisions of the people.
- With utmost effort I will attempt to keep myself well informed on advances in medical knowledge.
- As a socially conscious citizen, I will be alert to health hazards of the environment, join with others to eliminate such hazards, and do everything possible to advance the welfare of all the people.

These pledges may sound Utopian, and could doubtless be improved in content and scope; but I hope they convey a certain message. If the future physician is to be the "scientist and social worker" whom Henry Sigerist envisaged, a far broader code of ethics must guide his or her behavior than that which currently prevails.

But more important than a formal code of conduct that any person or association could compose is the need for the *education* of the doctor to awaken in him or her a profound realization of social responsibilities. In the 1980s, medical schools are still training physicians as though private, solo, medical practice were the norm everywhere. If the schools had heeded Henry Sigerist's plea 40 years ago, an ethical code on the social responsibilities of the physician would follow naturally; it would simply sum up the concepts of medicine that had been taught.

The social physician can no longer be regarded as an ethereal ideal of scholars and dreamers: he or she has come to be demanded by people everywhere. For health care is not like other goods and services in a community or nation. Inequalities may be long tolerated in the clothing, the shelter, the transportation, the recreation, or even the range of foods that a society allocates to its people; but for the direct preservation of life and health, nations at all points on the political spectrum must take action with sweeping social impact. The World Health Organization goal of Health for All by the Year 2000 dramatizes the special social status of health care. The medical schools of all nations must be inspired to train physicians who will be aware of the social realities of health and disease and of the doctor's place in the great social movements everywhere toward assuring health care as a human right.

REFERENCES

1. Sigerist HE: Medicine and Human Welfare. New Haven: Yale University Press, 1941; 145.
2. Badgley RF: Health worker strikes—social and economic bases of conflict. Int J Health Services, 1975; 5:9.
3. Flexner A: Medical Education in the United States and Canada. New York: Carnegie Foundation for the Advancement of Teaching, 1910.
4. Jonas S: Medical Mystery—the Training of Doctors in the United States. New York: Norton, 1979.
5. Fein R: The Doctor Shortage—An Economic Diagnosis. Washington, DC: Brookings Institution, 1967.
6. Mountin JW, et al.: Health Service Areas—Estimates of Future Physician Requirements. Washington, DC: Public Health Service, 1949 (Bulletin No. 305).
7. Terris M: Issues in primary care—false starts and lesser alternatives. Bull New York Acad Med 1977; 53:129.
8. Roemer MI: Primary care and physician extenders in affluent countries. Int J Health Serv 1977; 7:545.
9. Pflanz M: German health insurance—the evolution and current problems of the pioneer system. Int J Health Serv 1971; 1:315.
10. Roemer R, Roemer MI: Health Manpower Policies in the Belgian Health Care System. Washington, DC: US Health Resources Administration, 1977; 9.
11. Southby RMF, Chesterman F: Australia—Health Facts 1979. Sydney: University of Sydney School of Public Health and Tropical Medicine, 1979.

12. Roemer MI, Roemer R: Health Manpower in the Socialist Health Care System of Poland. Washington, DC: US Health Resources Administration, 1978; 24–25.
13. Myrdal G: Beyond the Welfare State. New Haven: Yale University Press, 1960.
14. Bowers JC, Purcell E (Ed): World Trends in Medical Education—Faculty, Students, and Curriculum. New York: Josiah Macy Jr Foundation, 1971.
15. World Medical Association: Declaration of Geneva. Reprinted in Reiser SJ et al: Ethics in Medicine—Historical Perspectives and Contemporary Concerns. Cambridge: MIT Press, 1977; 37.

Index